LEMONS ^{TO} LAVENDER

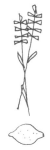

NATURAL REMEDIES BY
GORDON SAMBIDGE
ILLUSTRATED BY
KATE HEPBURN

For my mother, Grete Sambidge.
Thanks for all the support.

Text copyright © Gordon Sambidge, 1992
Illustration copyright © Kate Hepburn, 1992

Phototypeset by First Impressions, Lingfield, Surrey,
Printed and bound by Hartnoll Ltd. Bodmin, for the publishers,
Piccadilly Press Ltd., 5 Castle Road, London NW1 8PR

A catalogue record for this book is available from the British Library

ISBN 1-85340-123-4

Gordon Sambidge is a qualified homeopath and has a thriving practice
in North London. This is his first book.

Kate Hepburn lives with her daughter in North London. A graduate of
the RCA, her career has spanned across the film, music and publishing
industries.

AUTHOR AND PUBLISHER'S NOTE:
If symptoms persist or any remedy causes adverse effects, it is
advisable to seek assistance from a professional practitioner.

Neither the publisher nor the author is responsible for the efficacy or
suitability for any particular person of any of the remedies or cures set
out in this book. Whenever dealing with matters of health it is vital
that a proper diagnosis is made and professional advice is sought at
the appropriate time.

Introduction

This book is a simple guide to maintaining good health with basic methods and easily available natural remedies. It will help the individual take responsibility for minor ailments by finding effective cures within the home.

Health has a direct relationship to the quality of life-style, so by not abusing or pushing the body to a point of sickness, health will be maintained. This needs an awareness on all levels, mental, emotional and physical, ensuring each level is respected.

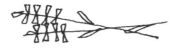

NATURAL REMEDIES

Good health is our natural state of being. The body constantly tries to maintain a steady internal equilibrium by regulating its temperature, blood-sugar and other variables.

However, our health is always being affected by external factors, such as stress from over-work, emotional upsets, or changes in climate and diet.

Any one of these factors can throw the body into a state of disorder. The body's efforts to compensate for these changes and restore the natural equilibrium cause symptoms. These come in many forms such as skin rashes, digestive problems, fevers or emotional breakdowns.

All natural therapies try to assist the body in restoring its equilibrium. They give the body energy and direction it requires to heal itself without suffering any of the side-effects often associated with artificially produced cures.

HOMEOPATHY

Homeopathy began with a man called Samuel Hahnemann at the beginning of the nineteenth century. Although its origins date from early Greek times, the first real structure of homeopathy was laid down by Hahnemann.

Homeopathy is based on the premise that "like cures like". This means that if a substance produces symptoms (onions cause burning eyes) in a healthy person, it will cure those same symptoms in an unhealthy person (e.g. Hayfever). Poison-ivy produces itching skin and inflammation but will cure those symptoms when given to someone with a similar skin rash, e.g. heat rash or eczema.

Homeopathic remedies are made from various plants, minerals, metal, animal products and human products. All remedies have been diluted, which makes them safe to take.

The amount of dilution indicates the strength or potency of the remedy. The most common dilutions are 6c and 30c; any dilutions higher than 30c need the advice of a practitioner.

Homeopathic remedies should always be used one at a time and never together. Remedies in 6c potency can be taken every two hours until improvement has been reached, then less frequently. The 30c potency can be taken every four hours for up to three days. They are taken in tablet form.

Homeopathic remedies should be allowed to dissolve in the mouth and no food or drink must be taken fifteen minutes before or after the remedy. Coffee and peppermint are to be avoided while taking remedies.

AROMATHERAPY

This is a method of treatment using essential oils distilled from various plants and flowers. There are about sixty oils with curative properties which have been used since Roman times; however, the term aromatherapy was coined by a French chemist, Gattefosse, who researched into the medical properties of oils in 1920.

Each oil has its own therapeutic nature and effect of the body.

Methods

MASSAGE is the most popular. The essential oil-usually around five to ten drops-is added to a base oil, and is received into the body through the skin, via a massage.

INHALATION. Place three or four drops of the essential oil in a bowl of boiling water. Cover the head with a towel and inhale the steam from the bowl. The oil can be inhaled directly from the bottle or cloth.

BATHING is very relaxing and therapeutic. Add five to ten drops of the essential oil to a bath, then soak.

NATUROPATHY

Most natural therapists believe that illness is caused by our bodies losing the natural instincts to exercise, eat, drink, and combat stress. Naturopaths recommend a return to a more natural life-style in order to re-establish the connection between body and mind.

The philosophy is based on the fact that the body has its own healing process and will return to health. This process can be helped with the correct guidance provided by naturopathy.

Methods of Diagnosis

IRIDOLOGY involves looking into the iris of the eye where various malfunctions relating to the rest of the body can be detected.

Methods of Treatment

DIET, by establishing the correct diet for the individual, eliminating harmful foods or substances, and introducing the appropriate nutrition to help rebuild the system. This often includes raw food and juices. There are also various mineral and vitamin supplements which help with organ and tissue repair.

HYDROTHERAPY, which involves the application of hot or cold cloths to the body to help fever or chill. This helps to regulate the body and aids circulatory problems in particular.

HERBALISM

Herbs have been used for healing in nearly every known culture in the world for centuries. Therefore a vast amount of information has been acquired about which herbs help which organs and functions of the body. Herbs can now be prescribed accurately to heal sickness. Recently, herbs have also been used as a source of drugs in scientific medicine.

Methods of Taking Herbs

INFUSION is the most common method. Place the herbs in a pot and pour boiling water over them. The usual measurement is a teaspoon of herbs for each cup of 'tea'.

DECOCTIONS are made from harder herbal materials such as roots or bark. Boil the plant material in a pot for ten to fifteen minutes and then drink when cool.

COMPRESSES are made by soaking a clean bandage in an infusion or a decoction and applying to the appropriate area.

POULTICES are formed by the direct application of the herb to the skin and applying a bandage. Often the herbs are macerated before being applied to the skin to ensure that rapid healing takes place.

TINCTURES are made by dissolving the herb in alcohol over a two-week period. Then the alcohol plus the herb constituents are decanted off to form the tincture. Tinctures are generally quite strong and should only have a dosage of five to ten drops.

Most minor complaints can be treated very satisfactorily by herbs but for more chronic conditions it is best to seek out a professional herbalist.

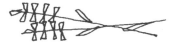

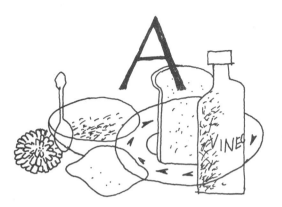

ABRASIONS

First wash cuts and grazes in warm water. There are a number of natural remedies which can be used.

CALENDULA (marigold) cream. Apply directly to the wound and bandage if necessary. This assists healing and is also an antiseptic. It lessens the chance of scarring.

HYPERICUM cream. Apply directly to wound and bandage if necessary. It can help with pain relief and nerve damage.

These creams can be purchased in a combined form known as Hypercal.

ABRASIONS

ARNICA 30c is a homeopathic remedy useful following an accident, as it can remove the shock factor from the system and prevents bruising. Take every two hours for the first day of the accident and then every four hours for two more days.

ABSCESS

An abscess is a localised accumulation of pus. It is formed as a protection when the body tissue is damaged.

SILICA 30c is the main homeopathic remedy. It can help to absorb the toxins of the abscess when the healing is slow, and is particularly useful for an abscess of the gums. This remedy should be given three times a day for three days. If necessary wait two days and repeat the procedure again. If it has still not cleared, or recurs, consult a professional health therapist.

HEPAR-SULPH 30c can be particularly good when abscesses occur on unhealthy skin and are sensitive to touch. It can help burst the abscess and drain out the toxins. It should be used in the same way as silica.

ABSCESS

BREAD OR POTATO POULTICES. These have been used for generations to draw out an abscess. A bread poultice is one of the most traditional: white bread is best. Break up the bread and mix with a little hot water or milk. Then apply this directly to the abscess and use a gauze and bandage to hold in position, replacing it every three to five hours. A potato poultice can also be used, either raw or pulped. Generally, a hot poultice has a greater drawing power.

ACCIDENTS

ARNICA (see Abrasions).

RESCUE REMEDY is a Bach flower remedy. A few drops on the tongue every half hour, can help with shock and traumatic situations.

ACIDITY

Chewing slowly and thoroughly allows digestion to take place at a more leisurely pace and prevents a large acid build-up.

LEMON JUICE is one of the best cures for acid digestion. Put two teaspoons of freshly squeezed lemon juice in a small glass of hot water and take in sips two hours after every meal.

CIDER-VINEGAR. A wine glass of hot water with a teaspoon of cider-vinegar taken in the same way as lemon juice, can also help.

SLIPPERY ELM can soothe and coat the stomach and intestinal walls, preventing any of the usual burning pains. It can be taken in a tablet form, or as a decoction.

CARBO-VEG 6c can help where there is heartburn and bloating of the stomach.

LYCOPODIUM 6c may be useful with acidity caused by nervous problems with abdominal bloating.

ACNE

GOOD DIET is extremely important to help clear acne. Certain foods should be avoided, such as white sugar and its products, white flour, fried and oily foods, chocolate, animal fats, and full fat milk and cream. Fresh fruit, brown rice, salads, and particularly apricots and watercress, are very good for the skin.

CARROT, GRAPEFRUIT AND CELERY JUICE is often beneficial for detoxifying the skin. It should be drunk twice a day.

YARROW ROOT DECOCTION, OR LEMON JUICE AND WATER can both make excellent face washes.

BURDOCK, DANDELION, ECHINACEA AND RED CLOVER TEA drunk twice a day for a month, may help.

The following remedies can be taken three times a day for two weeks. If there is an improvement on any one of these, then take the 30c potency three times a day for one day; then wait a week and repeat this once more. If the acne persists in causing problems consult a professional practitioner.

SILICA 6c can be good for pustules and spots with a discharge.

CALC-SULPH 6c may be used for multiple tiny pustules.

SULPHUR 6c can be good for hot skin with raised red spots and when the skin is worse with washing.

ACNE

KALI-BROM 6c is for acne of the face and back, especially before and during the menstrual cycle.

PULSATILLA 6c is for skin aggravated by oily foods and heat.

ADENOIDS

AGRAPHIS NUTANS 6c OR CALC-PHOS 6c can be taken three times daily for a week, if the adenoids are enlarged.

☦

ALCOHOLISM

Alcoholism is a very serious addiction or disease. It is crucial to seek professional help.

RAW HONEY can supply some of the nutrients lost with alcoholism.

ANGELICA ROOT TEA DECOCTION can help create a distaste for alcohol.

VITAMIN B taken on a regular basis may help repair the nervous system, which is often destroyed by continued use of alcohol.

ALLERGIES

Most allergic conditions need professional treatment.

CHAMOMILE AND YARROW HERB INFUSION can help soothe allergic irritations.

The following remedies can be taken three times daily for up to a week:

APIS 6c can reduce the reaction from stings and insect bites.

URTICA URENS 6c may help with heat rashes or allergic food reactions.

ANAEMIA

This is a problem of iron assimilation and absorption into the system, therefore the amount of iron ingested is not so important. It is caused by either lack of blood or a blood deficiency.

VITAMINS C AND B can help with iron assimilation.

RAW JUICES such as spinach, carrot, nettle and horse radish often help. This combination of juices should be taken three times daily.

ANAEMIA

The homeopathic remedies can be given three times daily for a week, and then repeated on a monthly basis if found to be helpful.

FERRUM MET 6c can help with pernicious (very severe) anaemia.

FERRUM-PHOS 6c OR CALC-PHOS 6c can be useful with iron deficiency.

NAT-MUR 6c can be useful when iron deficiency is accompanied by weight loss, palpitations and depression.

PHOSPHORUS 6c can be good in tall, sensitive people.

CALCIUM AND COPPER SUPPLEMENTS can be useful in aiding iron absorption.

ANOREXIA

Anorexia is mainly an emotional and psychological problem, and therefore it is necessary to seek professional help.

MALT EXTRACT in a glass of hot milk or water before meals can help build up the body.

ANOREXIA

KELP is a great normaliser of the body and so can help replace lost weight. It is taken on a daily basis in tablet form.

Both the following tinctures can be given in a small glass of water with five to ten drops of each, taken three times daily;

ALFALFA HERBAL TINCTURE can help stimulate the appetite and increase energy.

AVENA SATIVA TINCTURE can help deal with the anxiety and stress suffered while trying to stimulate the appetite.

ANGINA

This is a pain in the chest, caused by over exertion. This complaint needs professional guidance.

CRAETEGUS HERBAL TINCTURE can be taken on a daily basis to help relieve stress on the heart and circulation. It can also lessen pains around the heart and left arm. Five to ten drops of the tincture should be added to a small wine glass of water and this should be drunk two or three times a day.

ANTIBIOTICS

Over-use of antibiotics can deplete the body of its natural bacteria and leave the system empty of its own fauna and flora.

LIVE YOGHURT, LACTOBACILLUS TABLETS AND ALFALFA TABLETS can all help to restore the body's internal balance.

ANXIETY

CHAMOMILE, PASSÍFLORA, SKULL-CAP, LIME-FLOWERS AND VALERIAN HERBS can all act as calmatives and bring about a more relaxed state of being. An infusion of any one of these herbs may help, and a combination of teas may be even more effective.

LAVENDER, GERANIUM OR BASIL OILS. A few drops of these in a bath can help.

RESCUE REMEDY, the Bach flower remedy, can give immediate results in very anxious situations.

GELSEMIUM 30c OR ARGENTUM-NIT 30c can help when anxiety is due to a particular event such as an exam, interview or public speaking. They can be taken up to three times a day.

The following remedies can be taken three times a day for one day and then repeated the same way after a week:

LYCOPODIUM 30c can help with anticipatory anxiety with digestive complaints.

PHOSPHORUS 30c can be useful with anxiety concerning the dark, ghosts, health and robbers.

PULSATILLA 30c can help with panic attacks, especially of a claustrophobic type.

CALC-CARB 30c can be useful for real worriers who are anxious that something bad might happen.

ARSENICUM 30c can help for anxiety accompanied by restlessness and exhaustion.

ARTHRITIS

Arthritis is an inflammation of the joints. It is a chronic condition and generally needs professional help.

LOW ACID DIET can be very important in helping to regulate arthritis. Low acid foods such as raw vegetables, low acid fruits, salads, sprouts, brewers' yeast and wheat-germ all help.

ARTHRITIS

EPSOM SALTS baths twice a week can help draw out the toxins through the skin. Two handfuls of Epsom salts in a bath is enough.

ROSEMARY, COMFREY OR NETTLE TEA can help with the pains. Two cups a day is best.

CIDER VINEGAR AND HONEY in warm water, taken three times a day can soothe aching joints and muscles.

COD LIVER OIL either taken in capsules or rubbed into the joints may reduce the pains.

TOMATO JUICE, WHEAT-GERM, YEAST AND LECITHIN. Take four ounces of tomato juice, a teaspoon of wheatgerm, a teaspoon of yeast and a teaspoon of lecithin one hour before meals. This may help restore the acid-alkali balance.

These homeopathic remedies can be taken three times a day for a week; then wait a week and repeat the procedure once again:

RHUS-TOX 6c can help with the types of arthritis when the pains are worse sitting down and with initial movement, but become better with continued movement.

BRYONIA 6c can be good for pains that are better when pressure is applied but worse with any movement.

APIS AND LEDUM 6c can both be very useful for pulsatilla arthritis. This arthritis moves from place to place around the body, and the joints can be red and swollen.

ASTHMA

Simple cases of asthma usually respond well to a water and fruit juice fast for a few days.

RAW JUICES such as grapefruit, carrot and celery can help.

COLTSFOOT OR HYSSOP TEA can be good for clearing extra mucus and catarrh from the lungs, and also for aiding breathing.

These two tinctures can be given three times daily with five to ten drops in half a wine glass of water:

LOVELIA INFLATA TINCTURE can be excellent for all types of asthma.

GRINDELIA TINCTURE can help when coughing or wheezing comes on at night during sleep.

ASTHMA

These remedies can be taken three times a day for one day
and then repeated once more in a week's time:

ARSENICUM 30c can be good for short anxious breathing
with wheezing and restlessness.

KALI-CARB 30c can help with the shortness of breath which
occurs after waking from sleep and coughing up white mucus.

PHOSPHORUS 30c can be used for asthma with constriction
of the chest, anxiety and a thirst for cold drinks.

IPECACUANHA 30c can be used for inflamed bronchial tubes
caused by gagging from coughlng over excessive mucus.

ATHLETE'S FOOT

This is a yeast infection which occurs particularly.between the
toes.

CIDER-VINEGAR can be dabbed on the affected area morning
and evening till the infection clears.

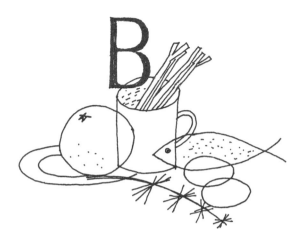

BAD BREATH

The common causes of halitosis (bad breath) are usually poor dental hygiene or bad teeth. Thrush infections of the digestive system and chronic constipation can also cause it.

PARSLEY, PEPPERMINT OR FENUGREEK TEA drunk once a day can all help.

CHLOROPHYLL TABLETS AND MERCURY 6c can also be useful.

BED SORES

Bed sores are caused by skin irritation.

Preventative: frequent changing of the patient's position and cushioning usually stops bed sores developing.

PERIWINKLE FLOWERS AND LEAVES DECOCTION applied to the sore may help greatly.

CALENDULA AND HYPERICUM CREAM in equal parts applied to the sore may give pain relief and healing.

⊹

BED-WETTING

Usually by their third birthday most children are dry at night. Those who continue to pass urine often do so for emotional reasons rather than physical ones, though a non-stimulant diet should be encouraged by reducing sweets and food colourings.

CHAMOMILE, ST JOHN'S WORT AND HORSETAILS TEA drunk twice a day, can help.

HONEY. One spoon at bed-time can help retain water and promote sleep.

CYPRESS OIL when mixed with a base oil and massaged into the child's stomach can help with relaxation and prevent bed-wetting.

Homeopathy can help greatly with this condition, though a practitioner should be consulted.

BELCHING

Belching is caused by poor digestion.

PEPPERMINT tea, or a strong peppermint can both have a good effect.

CHARCOAL TABLETS taken daily, can work very well.

CARBO-VEG 6c OR 30c can have an excellent effect.

BLOOD PRESSURE

Raised blood pressure can be due to various factors such as poor diet, emotional stress or inability to relax or exercise. Other factors include various arterial problems, cholesterol levels, and kidney or adrenalin imbalance.

DIETARY RESTRICTIONS. Advice is necessary to help restore the correct weight/height ratio. A reduction in salt intake and avoidance of all cooked and processed animal fats and sugars can help.

A HOT FOOTBATH at night can help with reducing blood pressure.

CELERY, CUCUMBER AND GRAPEFRUIT JUICES can all help lower blood pressure if taken daily.

RASPBERRY LEAF TEA AND STINGING NETTLE TEA can both be useful. Stinging nettle tea may help with the tone of capillaries and arteries.

SKULLCAP, CHAMOMILE OR VALERIAN are all calmative herbs. Taken as an infusion they may help with mental and emotional causes.

YLANG-YLANG OIL taken in a little honey after meals can help reduce emotional stress.

BLOOD PRESSURE

CRATEGUS TINCTURE is the most useful heart tonic and balancing agent for blood pressure. A few drops in half a wine glass of water twice a day will probably make a real difference to all circulatory problems.

MAGNESIUM TABLETS may be taken twice a day with food.

ALFALFA TABLETS can help strengthen artery walls, which in turn regulate blood pressure.

LECITHIN TABLETS can help with increasing numbers of blood cells.

BOILS

A boil is a small abscess in a sweat gland or hair root. Boils are a symptom that indicates the body is trying to remove toxins.

ECHINACEA AND POKE ROOT herbs are blood purifying agents and a decoction of them drunk as a tea for a week can help clean the system and prevent boils. Echinacea tincture alone, may work very well. Put five to ten drops in half a wine glass of water and take twice daily.

BOILS

GARLIC. A chopped garlic poultice may help draw out the boil and reduce inflammation and swelling.

LAVENDER, LEMON AND THYME OILS can help heal the area. Two to three drops should be put in a cup of warm water and dabbed onto the affected area.

SILICA, HEPAR-SULPH AND SULPHUR 30c are the main homeopathic remedies. Tissue salt of silica taken three times a day can also be excellent.

BRAIN FATIGUE

PHOSPHORUS is essential for correct brain functioning, so a diet high in phosphorus often helps stimulate brain performance. Fish, apples, caraway seeds and raisins are high in phosphorus.

SAGE TEA may help improve concentration; two cups a day is best.

KALI-PHOS TISSUE SALT taken three times a day may help brain fatigue and nervous exhaustion.

BREAST
(FEEDING, INFLAMMATION, ABSCESSES)

Breasts have the function of feeding babies to give them total nutritional support for the first part of life. All indications suggest that breast feeding is much healthier for the baby than other methods, as breast milk contains antibodies which increase the child's immunity.

RASPBERRY LEAF TEA can help prepare the breast for nursing and ensures sufficient milk supplies are available.

SAGE TEA can help dry up milk flow when the breast feeding has stopped.

WHEAT-GERM OIL. Four to five teaspoons of this daily, and regular exercise, may help sagging breasts.

GERANIUM, ROSE AND LAVENDER OILS can help inflammation of the breast. Put one drop of each in half a wine glass of water, and use a cloth as a compress with the solution.

CALENDULA AND COMFREY OINTMENT can be good for cracked nipples.

LAC-DEFLORATUM may increase milk production.

PHYTOLACCA 30c can help treat mastitis by reducing inflammation and swelling.

BREAST

SILICA 30c OR PULSATILLA 30c can help treat lumps and abscesses. However, it is important to seek medical advice first, to determine the nature of these.

BRONCHITIS

Acute bronchitis is the inflammation and infection of the respiratory tract. It can coincide with measles, fever and flu. There is usually a cough accompanying a fever, though generally a few days' rest in bed will clear it. Chronic bronchitis is usually due to repeated acute attacks. This involves a persistent cough, tight chest, wheezy breathing and a lot of thick mucus. Cigarettes and air pollution are strong contributory factors.

ONION. Boil up to two onions and place them between layers of linen or flannel on the chest.

APRICOTS can promote healing of the lungs and three to six daily help prevent bronchitis and asthma.

BARLEY cooked, and mixed with lemon and water, can help soothe the lungs.

PINE OIL. Mountains and pine trees have always been good for the lungs. The odour of pine resin can help breathing and sleep, so pine oil may be placed on the pillow before bed-time.

VITAMIN A found in alfalfa, parsley and watercress can help with bronchial problems.

COLTSFOOT, HYSSOP, LUNGWORT, THYME AND SAGE used individually or together as a tea may soothe the inflamed tissue and repair the mucous linings of the bronchioles. These teas can be drunk three times a day.

BRUISING

COMFREY, YARROW AND WITCH HAZEL herbs, infused and used as a compress can improve bruisings and swelling.

LEDUM 30c can be excellent for black eyes.

ARNICA CREAM OR ARNICA 30c are the best homeopathic remedies.

BURNS

Minor burns can be treated at home, but for more severe cases hospital treatment is necessary.

COLD WATER. The most important thing to do immediately is to run the burn under a cold tap for five minutes.

STINGING NETTLE TEA. Soak a clean bandage in the solution and place on the burnt area. Repeat this process daily.

ALOE VERA can be excellent for burns. A leaf from the house plant is squeezed out onto the burnt area for immediate relief.

HONEY is often applied to the burn to help with healing.

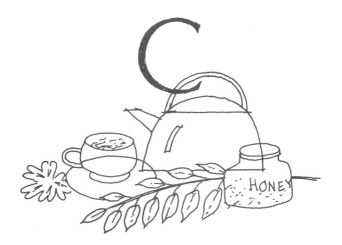

CATARRH

This is the discharge of the throat or nose, caused by inflammation of the mucous membrane.

DIET is an important factor to consider with catarrh. Milk and all dairy products should be eliminated; vegetables, fruit and salads increased.

COMFREY, GOLDENSEAL, BAYBERRY AND FENUGREEK TEA, mixed, can be drunk three times a day for up to a month. Put two to three drops of each in a bowl of hot water.

CREAM OF TARTAR. Half a teaspoon in half a glass of water can be taken before meals for a month.

CATARRH

EUCALYPTUS AND PINE OILS can be good for steam inhalations. Put two to three drops of each in a bowl of hot water.

KALI-BIC 6c, KALI-MUR 6c OR KALI-IOD 6c can be helpful in clearing catarrh and sinuses. Any one of them is taken three times a day for two weeks.

CHICKEN-POX

It is contagious twenty-four hours before the rash and remains so until the spots scab over.

CHICKWEED OR CALENDULA CREAM can help to soothe itching and prevent scarring.

LAVENDER, CALENDULA AND CHICKWEED combined as an infusion usually helps soothe the skin when cool and dabbed on with cottonwool.

PULSATILLA 30c OR VARIOLINUM 30c will often reduce the intensity of chicken-pox wonderfully, and shorten the recovery time. Either one should be taken three times a day for two days.

CHILBLAINS

Chilblains are usually due to poor circulation, causing burning, itching and swollen toes and fingers in cold weather.

HONEY OR GLYCERINE, EGG-WHITE AND FLOUR. Mix these together to make a paste. Place this over the chilblain and cover with a small bandage.

GINGER, BUCKWHEAT AND CAYENNE TEA may stimulate the circulation and allow blood to flow into the extremities. This tea can be drunk twice a day.

TAMUS CREAM, AGARICUS 6c OR PULSATILLA 6c can help. The last two can be taken three times a day for two weeks.

CIRCULATION

Poor circulation can produce a multitude of symptoms, so steps should be taken to improve it.

DIET RESTRICTIONS. Meat, animal fat, oils, dairy products and salt intake should be reduced, and a reduction in alcohol and cigarettes is essential.

EXERCISE is very important.

CIRCULATION

ALTERNATE HOT AND COLD SHOWERS help invigorate the blood vessels. Two minutes hot and two minutes cold for ten minutes a day often works well.

BUCKWHEAT TEA is usually good for building up and strengthening blood vessels. It can be drunk twice daily.

HAWTHORN TINCTURE can be excellent for regulating and balancing circulation. Take three drops in half a wine glass of water two times a day.

GINGER AND CAYENNE OILS may help if massaged into the skin with a neutral base oil.

COLD SORES

These usually occur at times of low resistance in the body or great stress. They may indicate an over-acid condition.

Preventative: Nat-mur 6c. Cleavers tea can be drunk in order to build up the immune system and prevent various disorders including cold sores. It can be drunk twice a day for a month.

BARLEY GRAINS. The acid condition of the body can be rectified by boiling barley grains for an hour, then drinking the water. This should be done at least daily for a month.

RHUS-TOX cream can be used directly on the sores.

COLDS
(see Influenza)

COLIC

This is a spasmodic pain in the intestines most common in babies and small children. Wind can be the main cause.

CHAMOMILE, CARAWAY AND FENNEL TEAS can help soothe the pains.

ROSEMARY OR PEPPERMINT OIL with a base oil, massaged into the abdomen, can be very soothing.

SULPHUR 6c, COLOCYNTH 6c AND CHAMOMILLA 6c can be wonderful cures if taken three times a day for two weeks.

COLITIS

Colitis is the inflammation of the intestines causing burning or spasmodic pains. It is often due to a stressful life-style or high anxiety.

DIET RESTRICTIONS. Certain foods will upset the digestive system, and these should be avoided, especially stimulants such as coffee, alcohol or strong spices.

MEADOWSEET, MALLOW, LAVENDULA AND LIMEFLOWER TEA twice a day can bring great relief.

FLAXSEED TEA taken ten minutes before meals can work well with the discomfort caused.

SLIPPERY ELM tablets or decoction, may help soothe the mucus lining of the intestine by making a temporary coating to ease inflammation.

COMPLEXION

WATERCRESS LEAVES AND TURNIPS are usually good for the skin, eaten in regular amounts.

CALENDULA TINCTURE, OATMEAL AND HONEY as a face pack, may be excellent for the skin.

LEMON JUICE mixed with equal amounts of water can be a good face wash.

CONJUNCTIVITIS

This is the inflammation and swelling of the mucous membrane connecting the eyeball and inner eyelid. It can cause the eye to discharge a clear or thick mucus or make the eye very red.

CHAMOMILE TEA, when cool, can be used as an eye wash.

EUPHRASIA (EYEBRIGHT), ECHINACEA AND CLEAVERS TEA is often drunk in combination with more localised treatments.

NAT-MUR 6c may be helpful taken three times a day for a week to improve the eye.

CONSTIPATION

If constipation persists, it is best to consult a professional therapist.

FIBRE. Constipation can be helped by a change in diet, especially by increasing the fibre intake, eg prunes, All-Bran, molasses, dried fruit and vegetables.

SENNA LEAVES, CASCARA, LIQUORICE, BUCKTHORN AND FENNEL TEA, in combination, can be drunk daily.

ALUMINIUM 6c taken three times a day for a week can help greatly.

CONVALESCENCE

After a long illness or cold, the body is slow to recover and is generally weak.

One of the following, taken every three days, can help:

CHINA 30c can be taken for two weeks.

GELSEMIUM 30c taken for two weeks, can help quick recovery from flu or a cold.

CORNS

This is a thickening of the skin, particularly on the foot, often caused by friction or pressure.

CASTOR OIL. Massage the corns with castor oil twice a day and eventually the corns will probably peel off.

WARM FOOT BATH WITH LEMON AND LAVENDER OIL can help peel off dead skin.

COUGHS

LEMON, HONEY, BRANDY. Hot lemon with generous dollops of honey and brandy can make a good drink to soothe coughs. Alternatively, honey, linseed oil and whisky can work well. Both can be used up to three times a day.

BYRONIA COUGH LINCTUS may ease very dry irritating coughs.

CRADLE-CAP

This is a series of small sores around the head which babies can get from lying down because of their very sensitive skin.

WHEATGERM OR ALMOND OIL. Rub on the baby's head and leave overnight. Then wash the baby's hair. Repeat this treatment when necessary.

CRAMP

This is a painful contraction of the muscles. It can be caused by cold, strain, or excessive use.

LEMON JUICE AND WATER combined can be drunk nightly to help cramp in the legs and feet.

SALT. A pinch of salt dissolved in the mouth before sleep can help night cramps.

PARSLEY TEA OR RAW PARSLEY are recommended for menstrual cramps.

CRAMP-BARK TEA AND RASPBERRY LEAF TEA can both be excellent for effective treatment.

MAG-PHOS 6c may be taken every five minutes during a cramp and every thirty minutes during menstrual pains.

CROUP

This is a hard dry cough which mainly occurs at night in children.

HYDROTHERAPY can be used by providing a steam atmosphere, either by boiling a kettle continually or by using a humidifier.

COLD COMPRESSES around the child's throat are good; change them when they get warm.

EUCALYPTUS OIL. Steam infusions of this can help ease the cough.

The following homeopathic remedies can be taken every hour.

ACONITE 30c can help if the croup is worse before midnight.

HEPAR-SULPH 30c can help if the croup is worse at midnight.

SPONGIA 30c can help if it is worse after midnight.

CYSTITIS

This is a urinary tract infection which leads to frequent burning urination. It can occur at times of emotional stress, when the body is very acidic, or because of a high level of sexual activity.

DRINKING EXTRA FLUIDS will help flush the kidneys and urinary tract.

BARLEY WATER made from boiling up barley grains can be drunk twice a day for a month to reduce the acidity in the system.

CORNSILK, COUCH-GRASS AND MARSH-MALLOW infusion, drunk every four hours, can ease cystitis.

CANTHARIS 30c drunk every three hours can work well to ease the symptoms.

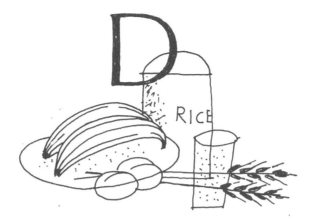

DANDRUFF

This is dead skin on the scalp.

ELIMINATE SUGAR from the diet.

VITAMIN B complex can help improve the condition of the scalp.

MILD SHAMPOO is recommended for the hair.

NETTLE TEA OR ROSEMARY TEA are recommended for the final rinse. Rosemary tea can help make the hair shiny.

VITAMIN E OIL may help itching of the scalp.

NAT-MUR 6c OR KALI-MUR 6c taken twice daily can help cure the dandruff.

 37

DEPRESSION

It is best to consult a professional practitioner for depression.

WHOLEFOOD DIET. This is generally necessary in aiding treatment.

VITAMIN B COMPLEX can help with a depleted nervous system.

ZINC TABLETS can help with neurotic depressions.

WILD OAT, SKULLCAP AND VERVAIN TEA can be used in combination. The plants used can work as nerve tonics helping restore calm to the body.

BASIL AND CLARY SAGE OILS can be good for massage or in a bath.

MUSTARD AND GORSE BACH FLOWER REMEDIES may be particularly helpful in lifting depressions.

DIABETES

This is a disease in which sugar and starch are not properly absorbed by the body. A professional practitioner should be consulted.

REGULAR EXERCISE is necessary.

DIET CHANGES. Lowering fat intake and increasing the carbohydrate content of the diet helps as this can reduce the body's need for insulin. Stimulating drinks such as coffee, tea and alcohol should be restricted. Fresh vegetables, fresh plums, whole grains, rice, lentils and bananas are especially good.

DIARRHOEA

This can be caused by various factors such as inflammation of the stomach and intestinal linings, food-poisoning, or stressful life-style and situations.

Preventative: ginger root in tea (water boiled for three minutes) can make a good prophylactic against infected waters in foreign countries.

APRICOTS. Three to five a day can work well in checking diarrhoea.

DIARRHOEA

BAYBERRY, MEADOWSWEET AND AMERICAN CRANESBILL TEA taken every hour until symptoms subside, can be good for acute attacks.

MEADOWSWEET AND LADY'S MANTLE TEA in equal proportions can be good for children's diarrhoea.

SLIPPERY ELM tablets or decoction three times a day, can help.

ARSENICUM ALB 30c OR MERCURY 3c can be taken every thirty minutes while symptoms last but for no longer than three hours.

DROPSY

This is the retention of fluids by the body tissues, causing swellings. This can happen all over the body or in localised areas such as ankles, wrists, fingers and abdomen.

JUNIPER BERRIES can help clear fluid. Boil five to ten berries in a pot of water, allow to cool and drink half a wine glass of it.

DANDELION TEA can be an excellent diuretic and should be drunk twice daily to remove excess water, though an increase in urination will occur.

NAT-MUR 6c OR PULSATILLA 30c taken three times a day for two weeks may be a great help in removing excess fluid.

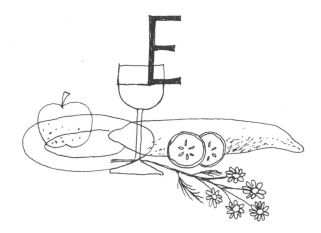

EARACHE

The eardrum is extremely sensitive to pain. It can become inflamed easily. Pressure of catarrh also causes the characteristic ache. Infection of the middle ear is indicated by redness and swelling of the outer ear.

HOT WATER. Placing the feet in a bowl of hot water with a cold cloth behind the head can bring good relief.

ONION CORE placed in the ear can help ease the pain.

SALT in a small bag, previously warmed and placed against the ear may ease difficult earache.

ALMOND OIL. A few drops, slightly warmed and placed in the ear via cotton wool often relieves discomfort.

EARACHE

MULLEIN AND GARLIC OILS can be very useful for pain and ear wax.

SILICA 30c OR PULSATILLA 30c can help with the catarrh in the ear and can be good for pain relief.

BELLADONNA 30c can be used when the ear is very red externally and it is throbbing.

KALI-MUR TISSUE SALT can be excellent for blocked ears and useful for plane journeys to stop painful pressure from take-offs and landings. It should be taken daily for catarrh in the ears and every twenty minutes before and during flight.

ECZEMA

Eczema is an inflammation of the skin resulting from an allergic response to an irritation. Its real root is inherited. Generally it is best to consult a practitioner for eczema.

RAW VEGETABLE AND JUICE DIET is cleansing and eliminating. It can help to clear the skin and bowels.

ECZEMA

CIDER VINEGAR dabbed onto the affected area can help contain the eczema.

CUCUMBER JUICE either dabbed on the eczema or drunk, can also help contain it.

RED CLOVER, DANDELION, MARIGOLD AND BURDOCK TEA taken three times daily for two months can be effective in clearing eczema.

CHICKWEED CREAM, CALENDULA CREAM AND E45. Chickweed cream is the best external application for eczema though calendula cream can also work well and E45 can help repair damaged skin and prevent dryness and flaking.

LAVENDER OIL mixed with a vegetable base oil can be useful when massaged into the affected areas.

NAT-MUR 6c may be useful for dry eczema around the hair-line and fingers.

GRAPHITES 6c can be used for weeping eczema which oozes a clear sticky fluid, especially in the skin folds such as the knees and elbows.

EYES
(see Conjunctivitis and Styes)

Eyes are wonderfully complex and sensitive organs and they can be especially prone to irritations, infections and strain.

EUPHRASIA TINCTURE is probably the most useful external treatment for eyes. It can help with sore eyes, blepharitis (inflammation of the eyelids), iritis and most other eye problems, by soothing and relaxing the eye and cleaning out any discharges or foreign materials. Place two or three drops of tincture into a quarter of a wine glass of water and then wash the eye with cotton wool soaked in this solution.

CHAMOMILE TEA when cooled can be used in a similar way to ease painful eyes.

CUCUMBER AND APPLE POULTICE can be good for swellings under the eye and inflammations of the sclera (pink eye).

RUTA 30c can alleviate eye strain when the eyes have been over-used from reading and detailed work. One dose can be taken every four hours for up to two days.

ACONITE 30c may be used when there is a pain from a foreign body in the eye.

NAT-MUR 30c can be excellent for dryness of the eye that can lead to iritis or pain. It should be taken twice daily for three days.

PULSATILLA 30c can be good for sticky eyes with a discharge which often occurs in young children and babies. It too should be taken twice daily for three days.

LEDUM 30c can be useful specifically for black eyes and will reduce the bruising and swelling quickly.

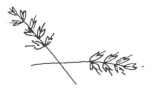

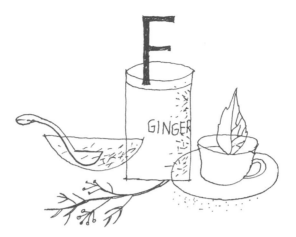

FAINTING

This is a temporary loss of consciousness due to the inadequate supply of blood to the brain. This can be due to low blood pressure, emotional upset, lack of oxygen, fear, or intense pain.

POSITION. It is important to keep the head lower than the body so as to restore the blood supply to the brain. Lift the legs when the patient is lying on the floor.

PEPPERMINT OR ROSEMARY OIL on cotton wool and held under the nose often helps regain consciousness.

FAINTING

The following homeopathic remedies can be given every thirty minutes for up to two hours after fainting:

IGNATIA 30c can be useful where the fainting has an emotional or hysterical cause.

PULSATILLA 30c can be used for when fainting has occurred in a stuffy atmosphere or crowded area.

CHAMOMILLA 30c can be used when it is due to severe pains.

CARBO-VEG 30c can be used when fainting is from exhaustion.

FEVER

This occurs when the body temperature rises above 37.2°C or 99°F. It is one of the body's defense mechanisms against infection. The increased temperature helps the body eliminate bacteria and viruses. If fever is very high and persists, it is advisable to call professional help.

WATER. It is important to drink lots of water until the fever has gone. It is best not to eat with a fever or chill.

TEPID SPONGING gives relief from the heat. This can be done using water or a mixture of water and vinegar. Only sponge one part of the body at a time, dry this area and then sponge another part. Keep all of the body covered except the area being cooled.

FEVER

ECHINACEA, CHAMOMILE, YARROW AND ELDERFLOWER
TEA can reduce fever and prevent infection. This combination
tea should be taken every hour during the fever.

The following homeopathic remedies can be given
individually every thirty minutes until improvement starts. If
there is no improvement after two hours, another remedy
should be tried.

BAPTISIA 30c can be useful for toxic fevers with a flushed face
and foul breath.

GELSEMIUM 30c can be useful for achey fevers with heavy
limbs and no thirst.

BELLADONNA 30c AND ACONITE 30c can be good general
remedies.

FLATULENCE

Gas in the digestive system is caused by air intake during
eating and drinking. Gas can also be caused by slow digestion
of food in the intestines or fermentation of food. Bloating,
abdominal pain, belching and passing wind are all resultant
symptoms.

FLATULENCE

Preventative: it is helpful to eat slowly, chewing food well and not drink during the meal.

ANISEED, CARAWAY, FENNEL OR PEPPERMINT TEA are usually excellent cures. They can be used as an infusion either individually or together, and are best drunk after meals or during periods of flatulence or bloating.

PARSLEY either fresh, or as an infused tea, can reduce gas.

PEPPERMINT AND ANISEED OIL. About three to four drops of each oil combined with a base vegetable oil and massaged onto the abdomen can work well in relieving tension in this area.

The following remedies can be taken every hour until improvement occurs if using the 6c potency, or once a day for up to three days if using the 30c potency:

CARBO-VEG 6c OR 30c can be good for bloating and belching in the stomach area.

CHINA 6c OR 30c may help distension in the upper abdominal area with no relief from passing wind.

LYCOPODIUM 6c OR 30c can be used for distension and flatulence with much gas in the umbilical area.

FOOD POISONING

This is due to the intake of food contaminated by bacteria or their poisons. Staphylococcus and Salmonella are the most common types responsible for food poisoning. Staphylococcus is found in dairy products or cooked meats. It releases toxins which cause symptoms for a short period of time. Salmonella occurs in a variety of foods, especially eggs. Symptoms include headaches, shivering, prostration, vomiting and nausea.

Preventative: Arsenicum album 30c taken once a week while on holiday can act as a preventative against general tummy troubles. Ginger tea can prevent poisoning from infected water when travelling in foreign countries. Add a slice of ginger to an ordinary pot of tea.

PEPPERMINT AND CARAWAY TEA may help settle the digestion.

The following remedies can be given hourly till the patient improves:

CARBO-VEG 30c may help poisoning when there is marked weakness, nausea, a pale face and diarrhoea.

ARSENICUM ALBUM 30c can be used for poisoning from spoiled meats or when there is food poisoning with colic-like pains from unripe fruits or vegetables.

FRACTURE

This is usually a break of the bone with pain, swelling and loss of movement. There are various types of fracture so it is important to seek medical help to ensure that the bone is set correctly before treating it. Wrists, ankles and collar-bones fracture most often. Old people are especially prone as their bones become weaker with age.

COMFREY is a major herbal medicine which has been used for centuries. It can encourage a speedy recovery of the bone. It can be used as a cream, drunk as a tea, or a poultice of the leaves can be applied to the break. It can also be used in homeopathic potency (although known as Symphytum), taking one 30c every three days.

The following remedies can be given once a week:

ARNICA 30c can help with bruising and swelling of the area.

HYPERICUM 30c may be used to repair nerve damage.

CALC-PHOS 6c, the tissue salt, can be given in daily doses when healing is particularly slow.

FROSTBITE

This occurs when the body is exposed to extremely low temperatures. It can affect fingers and toes especially badly. The frostbitten area, if not too severely damaged, can be revitalised by gradual warming at body temperature.

AGARICUS 30c can help heal the damage of frostbite and alleviate the burning and stinging pains. It should be given once every two days till the pains disappear.

FUNGAL INFECTIONS
(see Thrush, Athlete's foot)

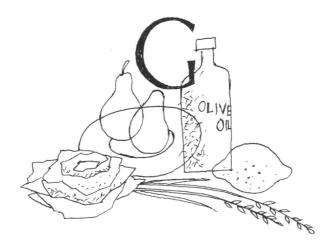

GALL-STONES

These are formed by deposits of excess cholesterol and are usually associated with inflammation of the gall-bladder. They cause great pain and discomfort if they obstruct the cystic duct. Those that remain in the gall-bladder cause no problems. Pain is felt in the area below the bottom right rib extending to the right shoulder.

REDUCE CHOLESTEROL. It is important to limit fatty foods and eat more fruit and vegetables. It is also necessary to stop drinking alcohol and taking too many stimulating substances.

CHAMOMILE TEA daily, can help break up gall-stones.

DANDELION TEA taken three times daily can help clean the gall-bladder and dissolve the stones.

GALL-STONES

EPSOM SALTS, HALF A PINT OF OLIVE OIL AND SIX LEMONS can help if the stones are long-standing and painful. The following procedure can eliminate the stones by allowing them to pass painlessly through the body. Take the Epsom salts first, then, one hour later drink a wine glass of olive oil followed by a small glass of lemon juice. After five minutes repeat this procedure until all the olive oil and lemon juice has been taken.

CHELEDONIUM 6c OR 30c AND CHOLESTERIUM 6c can be taken twice a day for a month to remove stones and reduce cholesterol.

GASTRITIS

Inflammation of the stomach lining is due to poor diet, excess alcohol, tobacco, or eating too quickly. Anxiety and stress cause an increase in adrenalin which releases stomach acids which inflame the stomach lining. Heartburn and acidity with belching and burning pains in the stomach are the usual symptoms.

SLIPPERY ELM POWDER OR TABLETS can help line the oesophagus and stomach which lessens pain with digestion.

MEADOWSWEET AND MARSH-MALLOW TEA can help with heartburn and stomach pains. Two cups a day should be taken.

GASTRITIS

ANISEED OR CHAMOMILE OIL massaged into the stomach area with a base oil or placed in a bath may give some relief.

One of the following remedies can be taken twice a day for three days:

CARBO-VEG 30c can ease the burning pains.

LYCOPODIUM 30c can be effective in gastritis where anxiety and stress are the causes.

NUX-VOMICA 30c may help when over-working, an excess of stimulants, and anger are the chief causes.

GINGIVITIS

This is the inflammation and bleeding of the gums, usually caused by poor dental hygiene or eating refined foods and sugars.

CALENDULA TINCTURE OR MYRRH OIL. Three drops of either, in warm water and used as a mouth wash, can help.

GLANDULAR FEVER

Glandular fever is an acute viral infection which concentrates on the lymphatic system causing enlarged and tender glands. This is accompanied by extreme exhaustion and weakness. This condition occurs frequently in adolescence and is sometimes called the kissing illness as the virus can be transferred through saliva. It is best to consult a practitioner for treatment as bad cases can last at least six months.

CLEAVERS TEA may prove of great assistance to recovery as it supports the lymphatic system. It should be taken three times a day.

VITAMIN C AND B, HONEY, GRATED GINGER, AND LEMON JUICE can all help.

GOITRE

A goitre is the enlargement of the thyroid gland, caused by lack of iodine in the diet or a malfunctioning of the thyroid. It is best to consult a practitioner with all thyroid conditions.

SPINACH AND CABBAGE JUICE can be drunk to help goitre.

KELP TABLETS taken daily can help.

GOUT

This occurs due to the build-up of uric acid crystals in the body. Uric acid is normally excreted in urine but with gout sufferers it gets deposited in small joints, especially the big toe, where the pain first starts. It causes swellings and inflammation of the joints plus pain on movement.

SIMPLE DIET. It is important to eliminate rich, fatty foods, stimulants and alcohol, plus red meat and acidic fruits. A reduction in weight usually helps.

GREEN CLAY POULTICE applied to inflamed joints usually releases toxins and absorbs them, which reduces pain and inflammation.

DEVIL'S CLAW TABLETS taken daily can be very effective.

BURDOCK, COUCH-GRASS, DANDELION AND SARSAPARILLA combined in equal parts as an infused tea, three times a day, can relieve gout.

LEDUM 30c, RHUS-TOX 30c OR BENZOIC ACID 30c can all work well. Any of these remedies can be taken twice a day for three days, then repeated in two weeks' time.

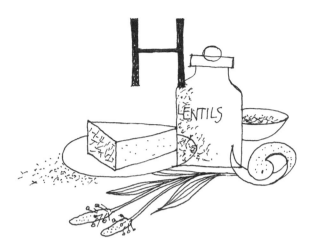

HAEMORRHAGE

A haemorrhage is excessive bleeding from blood vessels.
The flow of blood can be halted by compression on the edges
of the wound or pressure on the artery leading to the wound.
Tourniquets are best avoided but if necessary use a broad
cloth, which should always be released after twenty-five
minutes to avoid tissue damage. It is advisable to see a
practitioner when there is serious blood loss.

GOLDEN SEAL OR PLANTAIN are two herbs that can be
either directly applied to the bleeding area or taken internally.

CAYENNE in hot water can be applied externally or drunk to
stop bleeding.

CINNAMON TEA can be drunk to stop heavy uterine bleeding before other methods are used.

YARROW TEA drunk every half hour can help reduce the clotting time.

CHLOROPHYLL TABLETS also help the blood clot as they are rich in vitamin K.

GOLDEN SEAL AND WHITE OAK BARK can be used as a tea or in a compress around the wound. They can also be used as a douche or enema to stop internal bleeding.

MULLEIN. One ounce with two cups of milk simmered slowly and drunk daily can help to prevent bleeding from the bowels.

The following remedies can be given every half hour:

PHOSPHORUS 30c can be excellent in stopping arterial bleeding of bright red blood. It can stop nose bleeds, bleeding after tooth extraction and can help after extreme blood loss and internal bleeding.

FERRUM-PHOS 30c can also help nose bleeds.

CHINA 30c can be good after extreme blood loss and internal bleeding.

HAEMORRHOIDS (piles)

Piles are swollen veins which occur in the rectum. They may be internal or protrude to become visible externally. Piles can be very painful. They often rupture and bleed, especially while passing a stool. They can have a variety of causes, including constipation, pregnancy, poor circulation and liver congestion. Heavy lifting, and physical strain can bring them on.

RAW POTATO. A plug placed in the rectum with vitamin E cream can bring great relief.

WHOLEFOOD DIET especially raw foods, rice and pulses. Intake of sugar, salt and animal fats should be reduced. Coffee, chocolate and cola drinks can aggravate the piles and cause itching.

HAMAMELIS OR PILEWORT CREAM applied externally can help.

INFUSION OF GOLDEN SEAL, YARROW, PILEWORT AND WHITE OAK BARK can help reduce inflammation and irritation if drunk twice daily.

CYPRESS AND LAVENDER OILS in the bath can give good relief.

HAEMORRHOIDS

The following remedies can be taken once every three days for two weeks:

HAMAMELIS 30c can be used for piles with soreness which bleed profusely.

NIT-ACID 30c can be used for piles which feel like broken glass or sticks in the rectum.

ALOES 30c can help with piles which protrude like a bunch of grapes.

COLLINSONIA 30c can help when there is constipation and a sensation of sand in the rectum.

HAIR
(see Dandruff)

HANGOVERS

Excess alcohol causes internal dehydration and liver damage. Hangovers usually involve headaches, sensitivity to noise and light, plus general irritability of the nervous system.
If drinking is excessive it might be important to contact Alcoholics Anonymous.
 There are many types of headache and the more serious or

HANGOVERS

Preventative: it is always good to eat before a drinking session and take a vitamin B complex to help the nervous system. Nux-vomica 30c should be taken before going to sleep to prevent a hangover the next day.

JUNIPER AND BASIL OILS in the bath usually ease the tension of hangovers.

NUX-VOMICA 30c also can help relieve pain if taken every two hours in the morning.

YARROW, DANDELION AND BALM TEA can help the body detoxify itself after a night's drinking.

COCCULUS 30c can be good for nausea and vertigo after drinking.

HAY FEVER

This is an over-response of the immune system causing the mucous membranes to produce large quantities of discharge. It affects the eyes, nasal passages, throat and lungs. These areas are constantly trying to clear themselves of particles of foreign matter breathed in during the summer, which includes the pollen of grass, flowers and trees. House dust, cat hair and other particles cause a similar response.

HAY FEVER

EUPHRASIA TINCTURE. Put two to three drops in a wine glass of water and soak the eyes in this solution; it often helps stinging and burning.

EYEBRIGHT OR CHAMOMILE TEA when cooled can be used to bathe the eyes.

One of the following can be taken three times a day for two weeks:

ALLIUM CEPA 6c can help ease sneezing, watering and itching eyes.

ARUNDO 6c can help an itching palate and conjunctiva.

SABADILLA 6c is for excessive sneezing and itching nose.

MIXED POLLEN 6c can be useful for preventing the over-reaction to pollen.

NAT-MUR 6c can help a constantly running nose and dry eyes.

HEADACHES

There are many causes for headaches. These can range over stress, PMT, inflamed sinuses, high blood pressure, digestive or liver malfunction, colds, fever, sunstroke, injury, stimulants and muscle strain. There are many types of headache and the more serious or recurring ones should be treated professionally.

BAKING SODA AND LEMON. Take one teaspoon of baking soda and the juice of half a lemon in warm water, every fifteen minutes.

CLOTH SOAKED IN VINEGAR pressed against the head is a time-tested remedy for fever headaches.

MASSAGE AND FOOT BATH. A massage to the back of the neck and a hot foot bath can help frontal headaches.

WOOD BETONY, PASSIONFLOWER, PEPPERMINT, VERVAIN AND FENUGREEK INFUSION every few hours can help with most headaches.

CHAMOMILE, LAVENDER AND ROSE OIL in the bath, or massaged into the scalp or forehead, can help release tension.

The following remedies should be taken every half hour:

NAT-MUR 6c can help hammering headaches with misty vision.

SANGUINARIA 6c can help headaches which build up slowly and where there is vomiting.

BELLADONNA 6c can help headaches that throb with burning fever.

KALI-BIC 6c is useful for sinus headaches with pain at the root of the nose.

NUX-VOMICA 6c can help with splitting headaches with irritability and nausea, after eating.

IGNATIA 6c is useful for headaches which feel as if a nail has been driven through the temple.

HEARTBURN

Heartburn is a burning pain in the mid-chest area extending up to the throat and mouth causing a very acidic taste. There is usually inflammation of the oesophagus and backward flow of the acid content of the stomach. This can be due to a hiatus hernia or stress, fast-eating or poor diet.

ORANGE PEEL OR LEMON JUICE IN WATER taken a few minutes after a meal, can help.

MEADOWSWEET OR PEPPERMINT TEAS can be good if drunk three times daily.

HEARTBURN

SLIPPERY ELM TABLETS can help to line the walls of the stomach and oesophagus and prevent burning pains.

The following remedies can be given individually every half hour until the heartburn clears:

LYCOPODIUM 6c may help cure heartburn with anxiety.

CARBO-VEG 6c can help heartburn with a bloated stomach.

ASAFOETIDA 6c is often good for heartburn with severe belching.

HERPES

Herpes simplex is a virus which causes eruptions on the face and genitals. It often remains in a latent state around the nerve linings and may be activated when the body is run down, as stress and poor diet leave the body open for an attack. Attacks cause itching, irritation and burning pains around the genitals. The eruptions are like little blisters which bring much discomfort. The lymph nodes of the groin are often swollen when an attack takes place. It is best to consult a practitioner.

LYSINE. Intake of the amino acid, lysine, should be increased; it occurs in fish, chicken, milk, cheese, beans and fruit. It is best to reduce the amino acid, arginine, which occurs in chocolate, oats, wholemeal and white flour, peanuts and soya beans. Lysine supplements can also be taken along with an increase in vitamins B and C.

POKE ROOT, CLEAVERS AND ECHINACEA INFUSION taken three times daily during an outbreak can help.

MYRRH OIL in a bath greatly eases the discomfort.

NAT-MUR, SEPIA, PETROLEUM OR MERCURY 6c can help. Try one remedy every two hours during an outbreak.

HICCOUGHS

These are caused by eating too fast or by drinking too quickly, which brings air into the oesophagus.

HOLD YOUR BREATH for as long as possible.

DRINK WATER, hold it in the mouth and press fingers in each ear.

MUESLI. A teaspoonful of this usually helps.

HICCOUGHS

SAGE OR ANISEED TEA sipped slowly can help.

NAT-MUR 6c taken every fifteen minutes usually works.

HOARSENESS

LIQUORICE, SAGE, FENUGREEK, COMFREY, MARSH-MALLOW, MULLEIN AND GINSENG TEAS. The first two can work especially well when gargled, although the others are all helpful.

GRATED HORSE-RADISH, WATER AND HONEY mixed together and taken as a syrup can be very effective.

The following should be taken every half hour:

FERRUM-PHOS 6c can prevent or alleviate symptoms.

PHOSPORUS 6c can be good when hoarseness accompanies laryngitis.

ARG-NIT 6c can work for over-use of the voice from speaking or singing.

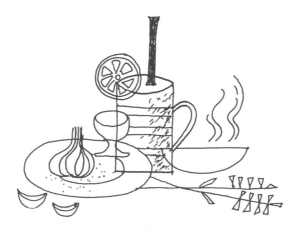

IMPOTENCE

Impotency can be due to exhaustion, and rest is recommended with no stimulants such as alcohol or coffee. Anxiety can cause, or exacerbate, the problem. Generally it is good to get professional advice.

GINSENG TEA drunk daily is suggested where impotency is caused and persists due to anxiety.

AGNUS CASTUS TEA drunk daily usually helps.

SELENIUM TABLETS, VITAMIN E AND KELP TABLETS taken daily can also be useful.

LYCOPODIUM AND PHOSPHORIC ACID 30c taken once a week can also help.

INCONTINENCE

Incontinence is common in old people, pregnant women, and people with anxiety and chronic illness.

MASSAGING between the third and fourth toes can promote blood flow to the bladder and kidneys.

AGRIMONY, HORSETAILS AND SWEET SUMACH MIXED TEA drunk three times a day, may help.

SEPIA 30c can help with urine loss from coughing, sneezing and walking during pregnancy. Given once and repeated a month later, it often proves very effective.

CAUSTICUM 6c can be taken for bladder weakness.

EQUISETUM 6c can be taken once daily for two weeks for incontinence and painful urination.

BARYTA-CARB 30c can be given once a week for a month to elderly people with weak bladders.

INFLUENZA
(see Fevers, Coughs)

Flu is a virus which affects people who are generally run down. It is the body's way of saying it needs a rest, and it takes time for the body to restore its energy.

Preventative: a mucus-free diet can help prevent flu so a limit on dairy products during winter is advisable as is a general increase in vitamins.

HOT LEMON AND HONEY is almost always very effective.

ELDERFLOWER, PEPPERMINT AND YARROW TEA drunk three times daily, can help deal with nasal catarrh and the aches of flu.

ACONITE 6c AND FERRUM-PHOS 6c can be taken if there is a slight feeling that flu might be approaching. These can be taken every hour for a day. They can deal with first stage inflammation and so stop the flu from developing.

EUCALYPTUS OIL can be used in steam inhalation to clear blocked passageways.

The following remedies can be given individually every three hours during the flu:

EUPATORIUM PERFOLIATUM 30c is helpful for flu with intense aching and bruised feeling.

INFLUENZA

GELSEMIUM 30c is the most general flu remedy. It is for flu when there are chills up the spine, heavy limbs and lack of thirst.

BYRONIA 30c is used for a flu with great thirst, aching on movement and irritability.

RHUS-TOX 30c is used for flu with restlessness, muscle stiffness and fever.

INSECT BITES

GARLIC can help to repel ants.

WET MUD placed on the area, can be useful for bee and wasp stings as it draws out the sting and controls the swelling.

HYPERICUM TINCTURE. Place two to three drops in an egg-cup of water and bathe the sting. It can help with the pain.

The following can be given every half hour while the pain lasts and then every two hours:

LEDUM 6c can be good for all stings and bites.

APIS 6c can help deal with the swelling associated with the allergic reactions to stings.

INSOMNIA

This is the inability to fall asleep or remain alseep for long periods. Anxiety, grief, worry and over-work may cause insomnia. If falling asleep is a problem then thinking backwards through the day helps induce sleep.

A HOT FOOTBATH before bed helps relaxation. Try relaxing each part of the body separately to relieve tension.

AVOID ALL STIMULANTS, especially coffee.

LIMEFLOWER, VERVAIN AND MARJORAM TEA can be good for promoting sleep.

CHAMOMILE, CALIFORNIA POPPY, HOPS, PASSIONFLOWER AND VALERIAN TEAS all help induce sleep.

LAVENDER, ROSE AND CHAMOMILE OIL in the bath before bed really helps.

AVENA SATIVA complex can help before bed-time by taking ten to twenty drops in water.

KALI-PHOS 6c every hour during the day for two weeks deals with nervous tension that builds up in the day and prevents sleep.

INSOMNIA

The following should be given once every three days for two weeks:

IGNATIA 30c can be good when vivid dreams wake the person.

COCCULUS 30c can be good for insomnia from a disturbed sleep pattern.

NAT-MUR 30c can be good for soothing activity of the mind before sleep.

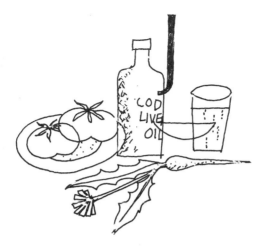

JAUNDICE

Jaundice indicates the congestion of the liver and build-up of bile in the blood. There is usually a yellowing of the skin and the sclera of the eyes, plus itching of the skin. This is a symptom of hepatitis so it is important to seek professional help.

TOMATO JUICE AND SAUERKRAUT JUICE. Half a cup daily can help clear the body of toxins and bile. A combination of various juices without food for three days can also cleanse the body. Continue until a normal colour returns to the skin.

CHELIDONIUM TINCTURE. Four to five drops of this in half a cup of water twice daily can be an excellent restorative tonic for the liver.

JAUNDICE

DANDELION ROOT, FRINGETREE BARK, BLACK ROOT
AND GOLDEN SEAL. A decoction of these can help the blood
and repair the liver.

CHELIDONIUM 30c OR CARDUUS MARIANUS 30c given
once a week for a month can be of great benefit.

JET-LAG

This can produce an artificial high, fatigue, insomnia and
dehydration. It can be especially debilitating with long-haul
flights, and air-conditioning and air pressure can irritate the
skin and dry out the body.

WATER. It is advisable to drink large quantities of water and
eat light salads, avoiding alcohol.

ROSEMARY OIL on a handkerchief inhaled on the flight or in
the bath after flying can help.

AVENA SATIVA TINCTURE can help the body recover from
jet-lag and eases the swelling of ankles during the flight. Ten
drops in half a cup of water should be taken hourly.

ARNICA 30c before and after flights can help the body recover
from the shock of transition and lack of sleep.

NUX-VOMICA 6c OR KALI-MUR 6c taken every hour during the flight can be good for the nervous system, irritation due to lack of sleep and general stress of flying.

KALI-MUR 6c can be good for the ear pain caused by take-offs and landings and this can be taken both before, and every hour during, the flight.

JOINTS

Most joint complaints need the advice of a professional practitioner.

COD LIVER OIL can help ease the pains and strengthen the joints.

MUSTARD OIL can help with stiffness and pain.

EPSOM SALTS. Stiffness in the fingers can be eased by soaking them in hot water with Epsom salts dissolved in it for fifteen minutes.

ACTEA SPICATA 6c taken three times a day for two weeks should relieve pains in the finger joints.

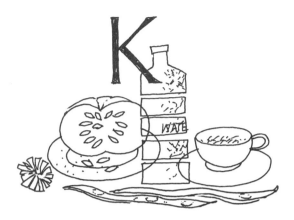

KIDNEY STONES

Kidney stones are formed by mineral deposits residing in the kidney. Stones are composed of calcium salts, oxalic acid and uric acid.

WATER. It is important to drink large quantities of water-at least six pints of fluid a day-to flush the kidneys.

NUTMEG, PUMPKIN SEEDS, CUCUMBER, DANDELION, GRAPE AND BEET JUICE can all work well to clean and repair the kidneys.

RUNNER BEANS eaten regularly are usually excellent for the kidneys and can also work for water retention.

GRAVEL ROOT, CORN SILK, HYDRANGEA AND STONE ROOT TEAS drunk three times daily can all work well.

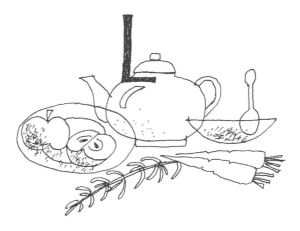

LABOUR

(see Pregnancy, Miscarriage)

It is important to consult a practitioner during pregnancy to ensure the correct guidance is followed for both mother and baby.

WATER. Fluids lost during labour should be continually replaced. The mother can suck ice cubes to help labour, or immerse herself in warm water to relax.

GOLDEN SEAL TEA can help strengthen contractions.

JASMINE OIL rubbed into the lower back after labour can ease aches and pains in this area.

LABOUR

ACONITE 30c can be given once a week, a month before labour when the mother is extremely frightened of the labour.

ARNICA 30c can help with post-labour pains and can be taken once every hour for a few hours then once a day for three days.

PULSATILLA 30c can help if the placenta is retained longer than half an hour after the birth until the placenta has been expelled. If this has not happened after two hours, medical advice should be sought.

PHOSPHORUS 30c OR IPECACUANHA 30c can help staunch post-partum bleeding if taken every fifteen minutes.

GELSEMIUM 30c can help cervix dilation. It can be taken one week prior to the expected labour date and every half hour if contractions have started with little cervix dilation.

CAULOPHYLLUM 30c can help contractions and can stimulate the uterus if there is inertia. This is given every thirty minutes during labour when necessary.

KALI-PHOS 6c can be taken every fifteen minutes for exhaustion.

LARYNGITIS

WATER AND VINEGAR. A handkerchief soaked in equal parts of water and vinegar placed around the throat can relieve pain.

RED SAGE TEA either gargled or drunk can help to ease laryngitis.

LEMON JUICE OR BLACK TEA can both help with the pain, as the tannic acid is a good soothing agent for throats.

LIQUORICE TEA can also help soothe the pain.

ARG-NIT 30c given three times a day can be taken for three days. It can be especially useful when the laryngitis is caused by over-use of the voice.

LIGAMENTS

RUTA 30c twice a week for a month can help repair damaged ligaments. It is used particularly for tennis elbow.

CALC FLUOR 6c taken daily for a month can help with elasticity of the ligaments, healing and flexibility in the future.

LIVER

This is the largest organ in the body and has an extremely important role in many of the body's physiological functions, including cleaning toxins from the body. It is important to eliminate alcohol and other stimulants when cleaning out the liver.

PARSLEY boiled in water for ten minutes and drunk three times daily can help with liver obstructions.

CARROT AND APPLE JUICE can also help with cleansing.

JUNIPER AND ROSEMARY OILS in the bath can help.

DANDELION, MEADOWSWEET, BURDOCK AND FRINGETREE BARK TEA can be an excellent tonic for liver if drunk after every meal.

CHELIDONIUM TINCTURE. Five drops in half a cup of water can be an excellent tonic if taken daily for a month.

CHELIDONIUM 30c OR CARDUUS MARIANUS 30c once a week for a month can give the liver a restorative boost.

NUX-VOMICA 30c often helps people who have liver related complaints from over-indulging in excessive eating and drinking.

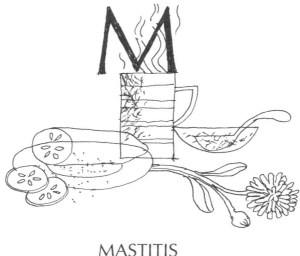

MASTITIS
(see Breast)

MEASLES

Generally a mild disease, the incubation period is one to two weeks. The first symptoms to appear are streaming eyes, nose, sore throat and a raised temperature. The rash begins on the third or fourth day around the ears and neck, extending to the rest of the body. Recovery is about a week later.

MARIGOLD FLOWER INFUSION drunk three times a day can help.

MEASLES

CHAMOMILE AND ELDERFLOWER TEA can be drunk or used as a compress on the skin.

One of the following can be taken three times daily for two days:

MORBILLINUM 30c is the best homeopathic remedy for measles and can be taken three times daily for two days.

PULSATILLA 30c is used when the measles are accompanied by a cough.

ACONITE 30c can be useful when there is a high fever.

MENOPAUSE

Menopause is the ending of the menstrual cycle. It can be accompanied by various symptoms such as hot flushes, night sweats and palpitations. There is often dryness of the vagina and soreness during urination.

In the UK the average age for menopause is fifty-one years. It can occur in three ways: the periods just stop; the cycle, while remaining regular, becomes lighter and lighter; or the interval between periods becomes longer and longer until they finally stop altogether.

HORMONAL FOODS such as cucumber, liquorice and sarsaparilla can help flushes. Sugar, tea, alcohol and coffee should be eliminated.

GINSENG TEA can also help with flushes.

AGNUS CASTUS, FALSE UNICORN, WILD YAM AND BLACK COHOSH TEA can help with this hormonal adjustment. It can be drunk daily till symptoms improve.

PASSIFLORA TABLETS. One to three daily may help ease tension and anxiety.

GERANIUM OR ROSE OIL in the bath can help with re-balancing the hormonal levels and tonicity of the womb.

SEPIA 30c OR LACHESIS 30c can be excellent for all symptoms of the menopause. Either one should be given once a week for a month.

MENSTRUAL PROBLEMS

These can come in many forms such as amenorrhoea (no periods), dysmenorrhoea (painful periods), menorrhagia (heavy bleeding) or metrorrhagia (bleeding between periods). Amenorrhoea often occurs in adolescent girls. It can be due to shock, emotional upsets, poor nutrition or extreme exercising or a hormonal imbalance. Professional advice should be sought.

MENSTRUAL PROBLEMS

PERIWINKLE, BETH ROOT AND AMERICAN CRANESBILL
HERB TEA can help staunch heavy bleeding. It should be
drunk one to two times a day throughout the cycle.

TANSY TEA can be good for bringing on late or absent
periods.

PENNYROYAL AND TANSY TEA taken twice a day can help
start a regular cycle.

RASPBERRY LEAF TEA AND CHAMOMILE TEA can both aid
cramps and stomach tension.

CHASTE BERRY TEA can be excellent for mid-cycle bleeding.

CINNAMON TEA OR HOT WATER AND CAYENNE PEPPER
can help heavy bleeding.

CRAMP BARK TEA as a decoction helps soothe cramps and
uterine tension.

CLARY SAGE, CYPRESS AND ROSE OIL is usually good for
soothing most menstrual problems. It can be put in a bath or
massaged into the abdomen with a base oil.

MIGRAINE
(see Headaches)

MAG-PHOS 6c taken three to five times daily can be very good for pains.

SABINA 30c, IPECACUANHA 30c OR PHOSPHORUS 30c at the end of the period can prevent mid-cycle bleeding.

⚮

MISCARRIAGE

Miscarriage is a natural abortion occurring when the body can no longer support pregnancy. The causes can be stress, anxiety, gynaecological problems, trauma, injury or poor diet. The first symptoms of miscarriage are bleeding and pains in the womb area. At this point professional advice should be sought.

Preventative: plenty of rest and relaxation in the first three months of pregnancy. Blue Cohosh, False Unicorn Root and Cramp Bark combined tea can help tone and relax the uterus to prevent miscarriage. Three to five drops of Viburnum prunifolium tincture in a quarter of a glass of water three times a day can help prevent it. Apis 30c, Sabina 30c, Secale 30c or Erigeron 30c can all work well.

MISCARRIAGE

LAVENDER AND ROSE OILS in the bath, can help soothe the body after a miscarriage.

ARNICA 30c taken three times a day often works well after a miscarriage.

BELLIS PERENNIS 30c can be taken once a day for a week after the miscarriage.

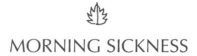

MORNING SICKNESS

Nausea and vomiting often occur in the first three months of pregnancy, mainly in the morning when the stomach is empty. Changes in hormonal levels, low sugar levels and low blood pressure are the main causes. Morning sickness serves to cleanse the body of toxic material, so protecting the foetus.

Preventative: meadowsweet, peppermint, ginger or black horehound tea taken three times daily can prevent sickness.

FASTING, SWALLOWING ICE, EATING YOGHURT OR DRY BISCUITS have all traditionally helped.

The following remedies can be taken three times daily for three days:

SEPIA 30c can be useful for nausea from food or odours.

IPECACUANHA 30c can help for vomiting without relief.

MERCURY 30c is for heartburn and nausea.

SYMPHORICARPUS 30c can be taken in extreme cases.

MOUTH ULCERS

These are small blister-like vesicles occurring on the gums, tongue, palate and cheek linings. Mouth ulcers indicate that the body is run-down and in need of rest. They can be caused by the over-use of antibiotics, flu, digestive problems, or emotional and nervous strain.

RAW JUICES, especially cabbage juice, are generally good for both the prevention and removal of mouth ulcers.

RED SAGE, THYME, OR MARIGOLD TEAS can be gargled or drunk separately or in combination.

One of the following remedies can be taken three times daily for two days:

MERCURY 30c can be good when mouth ulcers are accompanied by bad breath and excess salivation.

NITRIC ACID 30c can help burning and stinging ulcers.

BORAX 30c is for painful ulcers when the tongue has a coating. It can be especially effective for children.

MUMPS

This is an infection recognised by the swelling of the parotid glands or the neck. The incubation period is between two and four weeks. The symptoms start with a mild fever and sore throat with swollen parotid glands. Other glands can be affected such as the testes, pancreas and salivary glands. Mumps can cause infertility in men.

WATER, THYME TEA. It is good to drink large quantities of water. A thyme tea mouth wash can also help.

POKE ROOT, BORAGE AND ECHINACEA used as a combined infused tea is often an excellent tonic.

WATER COMPRESS WITH LAVENDER OIL in it can help soothe the symptoms.

The following remedies can be given three times daily for two days:

PAROTIDINUM 30c is a good general remedy.

MERCURY 30c can help when there is mouth odour and excess salivation.

PULSATILLA 30c can help when the person is tearful and thirsty.

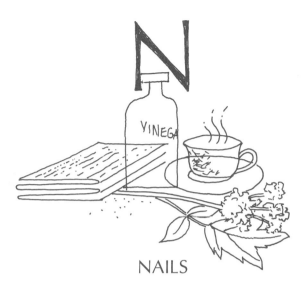

NAILS

They can break, flake and split easily.

EVENING PRIMROSE OIL can strengthen nails.

SILICA 6c can be taken three times daily for three weeks can strengthen nails.

NAPPY RASH

This is raw and tender skin around the nappy area of babies.

CHICKWEED CREAM, CALENDULA CREAM, WHEAT-GERM OIL OR VASELINE can all help.

PLAIN CORN STARCH dusted over the area can give good relief.

BICARBONATE OF SODA POULTICE placed on the affected area can help.

SULPHUR 6c, RHUS-TOX 6c OR MERCURY 6c taken three times daily for a week can remove the rash.

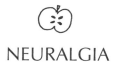

NEURALGIA

This is inflammation of the peripheral nerves of the nervous system. Trigeminal neuralgia and sciatica are the most common.

HOT SALT IN A BAG, BROWN PAPER SOAKED IN VINEGAR applied to the area, can help.

SKULLCAP, ST JOHN'S WORT, PASSIFLORA AND OATS taken as an infusion, can be an excellent nerve tonic.

NEURALGIA

SANDALWOOD OIL AND ROSEMARY OIL can be used in a bath or as a compress.

One of the following can be taken twice a day for two days and then repeated after a week:

SPIGELIA 30c can help trigeminal neuralgia with radiating pains.

HYPERICUM 30c can help with neuralgia generally.

MAG-PHOS 30c can help with sciatica and facial neuralgia.

NOSE BLEEDS
(see Haemorrhage)

POSITION. Holding the arm on the side of the bleeding nostril up in the air decreases pressure. Pinching the nose between finger and thumb and tilting the head back can both help stop the bleeding.

COLD COMPRESS on the back of the neck can help.

FERRUM-PHOS 30c, PHOSPHORUS 30c OR VIPERA 30c can be given every thirty minutes while bleeding continues.

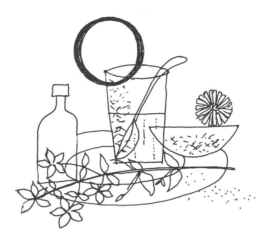

OBESITY

This is excessive amounts of body fat caused by over-eating, slow metabolic rate, lack of exercise or emotional stress.

KELP TABLETS for a short period of time daily can help regulate the metabolic rate and so promote weight loss.

PHYTOLACCA BERRY TINCTURE can reduce appetite. Take five to ten drops in half a glass of water twice daily.

LECITHIN TABLETS can help break down cholesterol deposits. Take one to two tablets daily for a month.

OEDEMA (water retention)

Swelling is due to the accumulation of excess fluid in the tissues of the body. This can be due to the kidneys not eliminating enough water, poor circulation, excess salt intake or low blood pressure. It occurs most commonly around the feet, ankles, wrists, fingers and abdomen.

DIET. A low sodium diet plus extra vitamin B complex can work well.

DIURETIC HERBS can be useful in removing excess fluid. Yarrow, dandelion or bearberry teas are the best. They can be drunk individually or in combination up to three times daily for up to two months.

One of the following remedies can be given three times a day, one day a week for a month:

PULSATILLA 30c is used for swollen ankles, especially in warm weather.

NAT-MUR 30c is used for swollen hands and fingers, with dry skin.

APOCYNUM 30c is used for general body oedema.

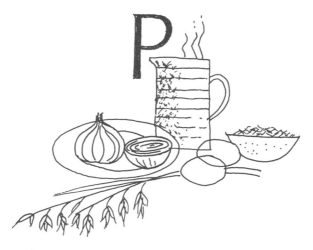

PAIN

This can have many causes, including injury, inflammation, disease or psychological reasons. It is experienced in the brain, so state of mind affects the severity of the pain. It is therefore especially important to relax and breathe deeply.

HYDROTHERAPY can bring good relief. Cold compresses may be especially useful for painful joints and sprains. Alternating hot and cold applications can work well with chronic conditions such as arthritis.

SKULL CAP, VALERIAN AND WHITE WILLOW TEA is often a good pain killer. It can be drunk three to four times a day.

CHAMOMILE AND LAVENDER OILS with a base oil can be massaged into the body for pain relief.

These remedies can be given three times a day for up to three days:

HYPERICUM 30c can work for nerve-damaged areas with characteristic shooting pains, especially fingers, toes and the coccyx.

KALI-PHOS 30c can be good for pain with nervous exhaustion.

MAG-PHOS 30c can be given for cramping pains.

CHAMOMILLA 30c and COFFEA 30c are for when the pains become unbearable.

PALPITATIONS

These are rapid and strong beatings of the heart, caused by factors such as stress, anxiety, fatigue, allergic reactions, anaemia and the menopause.

RELAXATION. Often with palpitations it is a question of just slowing down and having a more relaxed life-style.

MOTHERWORT, MISTLETOE AND VALERIAN TEA can be drunk three times a day.

PALPITATIONS

MELISSA AND YLANG-YLANG OILS added to the bath or used with massage oils can calm palpitations.

One of the following can be given three times a day for three days:

NAT-MUR 30c can help with a fluttering heartbeat and intermittent pains.

ACONITE 30c is used for palpitations with anxiety and faintness.

SPIGELIA 30c is used for violent palpitations with neuralgia of the arms.

PANIC ATTACKS

These are times of high anxiety which come suddenly and unexpectedly. They can be due to claustrophobic situations or crowded areas, though there are usually other underlying emotional causes.

NERVINE HERBS can help relax the system. Infused teas such as hops, valerian, vervain, chamomile and passiflora taken on a regular basis may ease tension and help restrict panic attacks.

PULSATILLA 30c can be good for panic attacks in crowded or stuffy situations.

PANIC ATTACKS

MERCURY 30c can work well with extreme panic and anxiety.

ACONITE 30c is used for attacks accompanied by a great deal of fear.

PLEURISY

This is an inflammation of the pleural membranes which line the lungs. It is caused by bacterial or viral infection and there may be sharp stitch.

LEMON JUICE. If there is a fever it is best to keep off solid foods and drink plenty of lemon juice.

FLAXSEED POULTICE. The flaxseed should be boiled and made into a paste. The poultice should then be placed on the chest and renewed every two hours.

One of these can be taken three times daily for three days:

BYRONIA 30c is used for pleurisy with intense stitch.

ACONITE 30c is used for a dry cough with burning in the chest.

SQUILLA 30c is used for shortness of breath and an exhaustive cough.

PNEUMONIA
(see Bronchitis)

This is a bacterial or viral infection of the lungs, which can be associated with secondary complications. There is usually fever, cough and sputum which can be bloody.

HOT LEMON AND HONEY frequently helps.

ONION PACK COMPRESS on the chest can help the inflammation.

POISONING

Hospital treatment is essential.

VOMITING. It is best to induce vomiting if poisonous material has been ingested. A teaspoon of mustard powder or baking soda in a glass of warm water will almost certainly bring it on.

EGG WHITES can help soothe the corrosive burning pains of poisoning.

CARBO-VEG 30c every two hours can help with nausea and pains.

POST-NATAL DEPRESSION

This can be due to exhaustion, hormonal imbalance, disappointment or weakness from breast-feeding. Counselling is always important.

AGNUS CASTUS, LADY'S SLIPPER, SQUAW VINE AND WILD OAT DECOCTION can help relax the body and rebalance the hormonal and nervous system.

BASIL, MELISSA AND CLARY SAGE OILS are often excellent for relieving the heaviness of depression. They can be used in the bath or in massage.

CIMICIFUGA 30c can be excellent for the inexplicable sadness that hangs around.

NAT-MUR 30c is used for general depression.

IGNATIA 30c is used for extreme distress with weeping.

PREGNANCY
(see Labour, Miscarriage, Breasts, Morning sickness)

Pregnancy is a time of great physical change as the body supports the growth of a child inside the womb. It is necessary to be particularly sensitive to personal needs and the needs of the foetus on both a physical and emotional level. A practitioner should be consulted during pregnancy as certain herbs and oils are best avoided.

GENTLE EXERCISE such as swimming, yoga, deep breathing and stretching all generally help to tone the body for labour.

NUTRITIONAL AWARENESS is important. Eat plenty of fresh fruit and vegetables as these clean the bowels and can therefore protect the foetus from toxins and body waste. The toxic effects of cigarettes and alcohol should be avoided.

CASTOR OIL can bring on labour if the baby is overdue. Drink three tablespoons a day.

RASPBERRY LEAF TEA has been used for generations during the last three months of pregnancy, to facilitate labour and ensure milk production. A cup should be drunk daily.

CAULOPHYLLUM 12c taken daily in the last weeks of pregnancy can help to ensure cervix dilation and easy labour.

PREGNANCY

A range of low potency homeopathic remedies can be used from the second month onwards. This is called the pregnancy programme and uses tissue salt remedies in 6c potency. Take two pills each morning and evening:

CALC FLUOR can help bone development, elasticity of connective tissue and may prevent stretch marks. This can be taken from the second month onwards.

MAG-PHOS is used for heartburn and nerve development. This may be taken during the second, third, sixth and seventh months.

FERRUM-PHOS is used for oxygenating the blood. It may be taken during the second, fifth, sixth and ninth months.

NAT-MUR can control fluid and salt balance, preventing swollen ankles. It can be taken in the third, fourth, seventh and eighth months.

SILICA is used for teeth, bone and hair development. It can be taken in the fourth, fifth, eighth and ninth months.

PRE-MENSTRUAL TENSION

This is the emotional and physical upset that occurs before, during and after the menstrual flow. Emotional disturbances can include depression, weeping, anger, irritability and anxiety. Hormonal changes can bring up emotions which are usually contained during the rest of the month. Physical problems can include bloating of the abdomen, swelling of the breasts, ankles and wrists, headaches, spots, nausea and vomiting, exhaustion, weakness and restlessness. It is best to consult a practitioner.

VALERIAN AND SKULL-CAP INFUSION can help anxiety.

CRAMP BARK can help with uterine pains.

DANDELION TEA can help to eliminate excess fluids around the body to reduce swellings.

EVENING PRIMROSE OIL can be extremely useful if taken before the period.

One of the following remedies can be taken three times a day two days before the flow is expected:

LACHESIS 30c can be good for anger, irritability and tension.

SEPIA 30c can help with headaches, nausea and depression.

NAT-MUR 30c can help with sadness, swollen ankles and water retention.

PRICKLY HEAT

This is a heat rash caused by blocked sweat glands during hot weather. It can be exacerbated by excess alcohol.

COLD COMPRESSES AND SHOWERS are usually helpful.

CHICKWEED CREAM can be applied to the problem area.

NAT-MUR 30c taken three times a day for three days can prevent or help it.

PROLAPSE

This is the descent of any organ from its normal position in the body. The womb, rectum and bladder are the most common organs to prolapse.

EXERCISE. Swimming, yoga and pelvic floor exercises, as well as general weight loss, can all help strengthen the body to hold the organs in place.

These remedies can be taken twice a day for two days:

SEPIA 30c can help for prolapse of the womb.

RUTA 30c can help a prolapse of the rectum.

PROSTATE

Enlargement of the prostate is a common problem for men in later life. It can be very difficult to urinate and residual urine in the bladder can become infected.

RAW ONIONS AND ZINC SUPPLEMENTS can help the prostate, as it needs a high zinc level to function well.

PUMPKIN SEEDS can help. Up to a pound a day can be eaten.

HORSETAILS, COUCH-GRASS AND SAW PALMETTO TEAS can improve urination and soothe the prostate.

SABAL SERRULATA TINCTURE. Ten to twenty drops in a wine glass of water before meals can have an extremely beneficial effect.

CAUSTICUM 30c once a week can help with bladder weakness.

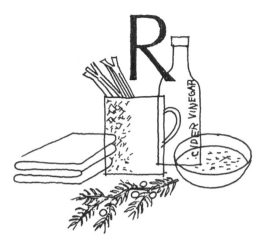

RADIATION

After radiation treatment the body may suffer various unpleasant side-effects.

RADIUM BROMIDE 30c can reduce these side-effects. Take once daily for a week and then repeat for another week after a week's break.

RHEUMATISM
(see Arthritis)

This is the chronic inflammation of connective tissue, usually fibrous around joints. The usual symptoms include pain, swelling, heat and stiffness in the wrist, elbows, knees and other joints. There are many causes such as stress, genetic reasons, an inability to eliminate toxins and poor digestive assimilation. Generally, it should be treated by a practitioner.

DIET. All rheumatics should pay great attention to diet-see Arthritis.

HOT EPSOM SALTS BATHS twice a week can be taken to ease the discomfort.

FRESH GINGER ROOT POULTICE can help the pains and swelling.

DEVIL'S CLAW DECOCTION may be drunk three times daily.

BOGBEAN, MEADOWSWEET, YARROW AND CELERY COMBINED TEA can cleanse toxins from the body and helps with the inflammation.

JUNIPER OIL can be useful either in the bath or as a compress.

RHEUMATISM

LAVENDER, ROSEMARY AND MARJORAM OILS added to a massage oil frequently help to ease the pain.

One of these remedies can be given twice daily for three days, then repeat this procedure after two weeks:

RHUS-TOX 30c can help with rheumatic stiffness and swelling, especially when pains are worse on first motion, after rest and in damp weather.

BRYONIA 30c can be helpful when there is redness, swelling and pain with movement, but when the pain improves if pressure is applied on the area.

APIS 30c is useful for redness, swelling, heat and restlessness.

PULSATILLA 30c is helpful for when the pains move from joint to joint.

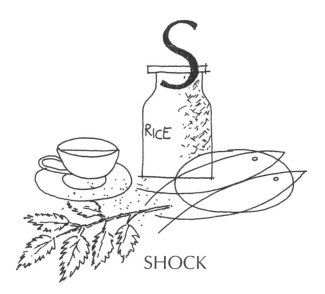

SHOCK

Shock occurs after injuries, burns, fright, blood loss or emotional upset. Signs include a fast pulse, pale face, nausea, restlessness and anxiety, all of which can lead to fainting.

LIE DOWN with legs raised to allow blood to flow to the brain.

RESCUE REMEDY can be taken every ten minutes.

CHAMOMILE OR SKULLCAP TEA can release the shock.

MELISSA OR PEPPERMINT OILS held under the nose can help.

ARNICA 30c every half hour after a shock can help. It should be taken until the shocked state improves.

SHOCK

The following can be given every hour for three hours:

ACONITE 30c is used for fear with shock.

IGNATIA 30c is used for emotional shock.

CHINA 30c is used for shock with great loss of blood.

✙

SINUSITIS

This is inflammation of the mucous membranes lining the nose and connecting sinus passageways. The nasal cavity can be obstructed due to colds, flu or hay fever.

REDUCE DAIRY PRODUCTS as this can help to reduce the amount of catarrh.

GARLIC AND PARSLEY taken every day often help clear sinuses during acute attacks.

FENUGREEK TEA is a good general remedy.

BAYBERRY, GOLDEN SEAL AND BRIGHAM TEA makes a good infusion which can ease congestion.

EUCALYPTUS OR PINE OIL added to a steam inhalation may help to clear the passageways.

SINUSITIS

One of these remedies can be given three times daily for three days:

KALI-BIC 30c is used for sinusitis with pain at the root of the nose.

ARSENICUM ALB 30c is used for obstruction with a watery discharge.

THUJA 30c is used for sinusitis with post-nasal and green discharge.

SLEEPLESSNESS
(see Insomnia)

SORE THROAT
(see Tonsillitis)

This is an infection of the pharynx and tonsils. It can be accompanied by fever, earache, and swollen glands. Sore throats indicate that the body is run down, so rest and fresh foods, plus plenty of fluids, are important.

WARM SALT GARGLE can work well to ease inflammation.

SORE THROAT

FENUGREEK, HOREHOUND AND MARSH-MALLOW TEA, RED SAGE, ECHINACEA OR POKE ROOT TEAS drunk or gargled, can work well.

HONEY AND LEMON usually soothes the throat.

ALOE VERA JUICE in water can ease the pains.

FERRUM-PHOS 6c or ACONITE 6c can be given at the first sign of a sore throat developing. They can deal with the first stage of inflammation and should be given every hour.

One of these remedies can be given three times a day for two days:

PHYTOLACCA 30c is used for throats with swollen glands and pain on swallowing.

BELLADONNA 30c is used for a red, inflamed throat, with fever.

MERCURY 30c is used when there are swollen glands, foul breath and increased salivation.

LACHESIS 30c is used when there is pain on swallowing and a sensation of a lump in the throat.

SPLEEN

FISH, BROWN RICE DIET can help clean the system and rejuvenate the spleen.

BAYBERRY, DANDELION OR YELLOW DOCK TEA can help an enlarged spleen.

EUCALYPTUS OIL rubbed into the abdomen with a massage oil can be very useful.

CEANOTHUS AMER 30c taken once a week for a month helps.

SPLINTERS

These should be removed as quickly as possible to prevent infection.

CALENDULA CREAM can be good after the splinters have been removed.

SILICA 30c taken twice daily for three days will usually push the splinter out if it is embedded deeply.

SPRAIN

This is the tearing or stretching of ligaments which cause swelling and bruising. Ankles, wrists and knees are the most common areas to be sprained.

COLD WATER COMPRESS can help. Bandaging it on gives support to the damage while it heals.

COMFREY TEA taken daily can help healing.

RUTA CREAM OR RHUS-TOX CREAM can be applied externally to help muscle strain.

RUTA 30c is the best homeopathic remedy for sprains, especially tennis elbow. It may be given three times daily for three days, and then repeated once weekly until healing is complete.

ARNICA 30c can be given once daily for a week to reduce bruising.

STINGS
(see Insect bites)

STOMACH ULCERS

These are due to a portion of stomach lining being eroded by digestive juices. It can be caused by stress, anxiety, emotional upsets, poor diet, eating too quickly, smoking or alcohol. There are usually burning pains, griping pains, heartburn and nausea.

RAW JUICES such as cucumber, carrot, parsley or celery may heal the ulcer. A three-day fast with just juices can be especially useful. Spicy and highly-seasoned foods should be avoided.

MARSH-MALLOW OR MEADOWSWEET TEA can ease the pain and speeds up the repair of the stomach lining.

SLIPPERY ELM TABLETS can coat and soothe the stomach lining and so protect the ulcer. They should be taken twice daily.

One of these can be given twice daily on one day a week, for four weeks:

LYCOPODIUM 30c is used when there is anxiety and stress aggravating the ulcer.

CARBO-VEG 30c is used for burning pains with eructations.

STRETCH MARKS

Preventative: after bathing, the body can be massaged with sesame seed oil or wheat-germ oil to prevent marks caused by weight loss, pregnancy and scarring. Calc fluor 6c taken twice daily for a month can help skin elasticity and so prevent stretch marks.

STROKES

These are sudden interferences with the cirulation of the blood to the brain, resulting in some degree of muscle impairment to the body. Obviously it is important to consult a professional practitioner.

ARNICA 30c taken every day for two weeks, can help restore functioning, remove the shock and aid circulation.

STYES

These occur in the follicle of the eyelash due to bacterial infection. This occurs when the body is run-down and lacking energy.

STYES

RESTRICTED DIET. It is best to avoid eating eggs, fish and chicken when styes occur.

VITAMIN B complex can be useful to improve the nervous system.

CHAMOMILE TEA can be used as an eye-wash.

EUPHRASIA TINCTURE can be a good eye-wash. Put three to five drops in a quarter of a glass of water, and wash the eye three times a day.

The following can be given three times daily for two days.

STAPHYAGRIA 30c is used for recurrent styes.

SILICA 30c is used if the stye shows no sign of discharging.

☥

SUNBURN

This is over-exposure to the ultra-violet rays of the sun, which causes redness, tenderness and blistering of the skin.

WATER. Cool the body in water and drink lots of fluids. After cooling the body, try to avoid chill by wearing warm clothes and avoid future exposure to the sun until the skin has healed.

NETTLE TEA drunk three times daily or used as a compress can work very well.

CALENDULA CREAM or HOMEOPATHIC BURNS CREAM can be applied directly.

ALOE VERA GEL applied directly to the skin can reduce the pains.

CANTHARIS 30c taken after a day in the sun can reduce the risk of burning. If the skin is severely burned, it should be taken three times daily for two days.

SUNSTROKE

This can cause vomiting, nausea, weakness and a pounding headache.

FLUIDS should be drunk to help the body with dehydration.

Either of these remedies can be taken three times daily for a day:

BELLADONNA 30c can be given with sunstroke plus a pounding headache and great body heat.

CARBO-VEG 30c can be used for sunstroke with collapse, nausea and a pale face.

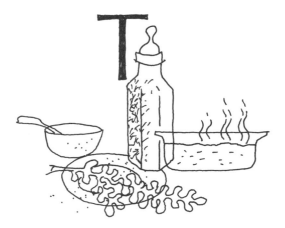

TEETHING

This is the soreness and irritation experienced by babies as their new teeth push through the gums. The pain can be accompanied by fever, flushed cheeks, diarrhoea and extreme irritability.

OLIVE OIL rubbed on the gums, can soothe them.

CHAMOMILE can be taken, either as a tea in the baby's bottle, or as a homeopathic remedy, Chamomilla 30c every two hours for up to two days.

CALC FLUOR 6c given once a day for a month can strengthen the enamel in weak teeth.

TENNIS ELBOW
(see Sprain)

THRUSH (Candida)

This is an infection due to a yeast-like fungus called Candida albicans. The yeast occurs naturally in the bowel area, though during stressful times this level can increase greatly. Over-use of antibiotics, fatigue, a weakened immune system and a poor diet can also be responsible. Thrush can occur in the mouth, bowel or vagina.

RESTRICTED DIET. It is important to have a diet free of sugar, starch and wheat products.

CIDER VINEGAR can be excellent in curing thrush. A tablespoon a day returns the body to a more acidic level in which a yeast fungus cannot survive.

LACTOBACILLUS ACIDOPHILUS SUPPLEMENT may be taken daily. This can replace the bacteria that control the growth of thrush.

BORAX 30c can help thrush of the mouth, especially in babies. It should be given three times daily for two days.

THYROID

This is an important gland that controls metabolic rates and the menstrual cycle. It is best to consult a practitioner.

IODINE. The thyroid needs a high level of iodine to function well. It can be ingested in seaweed or kelp tablets on a daily basis to help rebalance the thyroid.

BUGLEWEED TEA taken three times daily can help an over-active thyroid.

BLADDERWRACK TEA taken in the same way can help an under-active thyroid.

TINNITUS

This is a ringing and buzzing in the ear. It can be caused by catarrh in the Eustachian tubes, damage to the auditory nerve, or over-use of antibiotics.

GOLDEN SEAL AND BLACK COHOSH TEAS can help clear the catarrh and stop the noises for tinnitus which is caused by catarrhal blockage.

SALICYLIC ACID 6c taken three times a day for two weeks can help.

These should be taken twice a day for three days:

PULSATILLA 30c can clear the ears.

CHINA-SULPH 30c can help tinnitus with vertigo.

TONSILLITIS

Inflammation of the tonsils, especially in small children, usually due to a Streptococcus bacterial infection. This causes a fever and a painful throat.

BARYTA-CARB 30c taken twice a day for two days can help recurrent tonsillitis.

TOOTHACHE

HOT WATER. Bathing the face and neck in hot water can relieve pains.

CLOVE OIL placed on the painful tooth often works immediately in easing pain.

TOOTHACHE

HYPERICUM 30c every three hours for two days can help nerve pain.

ARNICA 30c for any injury to the teeth should be taken three times a day for three days. If taken half an hour before and half an hour after a visit to the dentist, it should make the experience less traumatic.

ACONITE 30c taken an hour before a visit to the dentist, can also make it less traumatic.

TRAVEL SICKNESS

Symptoms include nausea, vertigo, vomiting and anxiety.

POWDERED GINGER OR GINGER TEA can help during travelling.

PEPPERMINT OIL AND MELISSA OIL can prevent and ease sickness.

The following should be taken before, and every two hours during, the journey:

COCCULUS 30c can help travel sickness with vertigo.

TABACUM 30c is helpful for severe nausea with travel sickness.

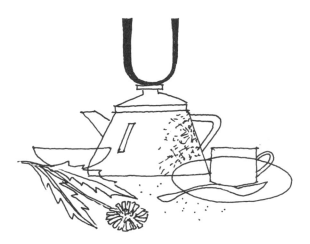

URINARY RETENTION

Urine retention is common in children and the inability to empty the bladder fully can lead to infection. Urinary problems such as discoloration or infection should be checked by a professional practitioner.

DANDELION OR YARROW TEAS can promote urination. Drink every day for a month.

Try one of these three times a day for two days:

APIS 30c can help for urine retention with restlessness.

ACONITE 30c is for retention with fever.

CANTHARIS 30c can be good when there is burning urination in small amounts.

 125

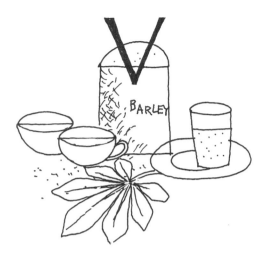

VARICOSE VEINS

Varicose veins can be caused by lack of exercise, pregnancy, obesity, constipation or water retention. The veins stretch and swell due to the back pressure of blood on their thin walls.

EXERCISE. It is essential to take exercise. Raise the legs after sitting or standing a long while.

WATER TREATMENT is good to stimulate circulation with short periods of exposure to hot and cold water alternately.

STROKING the veins upwards helps the blood flow back to the heart.

VARICOSE VEINS

WHOLEFOOD DIET is important, plus avoidance of alcohol and cigarettes.

DANDELION AND YARROW TEAS can help water retention and ease the pressure on veins.

HAMAMELIS as a cream can be applied externally, or can be used as a poultice to help reduce the varicose veins. It can also be taken homeopathically in 6c dosage, twice daily for two weeks, then repeated after two weeks. This should help circulation.

RUTIN can help strengthen the vein walls. It can be taken as a supplement or in buckwheat.

HORSE CHESTNUT, CAYENNE, GINGER AND PRICKLY ASH BARK drunk as an infused tea daily, can stimulate circulation.

CYPRESS OIL, SWEET ALMOND OIL in combination with a base oil and massaged into the legs, can help.

PULSATILLA 30c taken once a week for a month, can help sluggish circulation with cold feet.

CALC FLUOR 6c can improve elasticity of the walls and contracts the veins.

VERTIGO

This is dizziness, associated with the impression that oneself or one's surroundings are rotating. Nausea, headache, and vomiting accompany vertigo. It is caused by disturbance in the balance mechanism of the inner ear, or a disturbance of the auditory nerve.

COCCULUS 30c can be excellent for vertigo with nausea and palpitations.

CONIUM 30c is for vertigo while lying down or turning over in bed.

PULSATILLA 30c is for vertigo with fainting when looking up or down.

GELSEMIUM 30c is for dizziness after an exhaustive flu or illness.

VOMITING

Nausea, sweating, a pale face and tachycardia are all symptoms leading to vomiting. There are many causes such as shock, pregnancy, food or alcohol poisoning, unpleasant odours, emotional upsets, vertigo and head injury.

VOMITING

FASTING is a good way to reduce vomiting.

SLIPPERY ELM TABLETS can help line the stomach wall and ease the vomiting.

SWALLOWING CRACKED ICE can reduce vomiting.

BARLEY boiled and simmered for ten minutes in two cups of water and drunk, can ease vomiting.

MEADOWSWEET TEA can alleviate nausea and controls vomiting.

PEPPERMINT OIL plus a base oil massaged into the tummy can ease the vomiting.

One of these remedies can be given three times a day for two days:

IPECACUANHA 30c is for vomiting with nausea.

ARSENICUM ALB 30c is for vomiting accompanied by a burning sensation and diarrhoea.

NUX-VOMICA 30c is for the violent vomiting of bilious, sour vomit due to over-indulgence in food or alcohol.

AETHUSA 30c is given to babies vomiting their mother's milk.

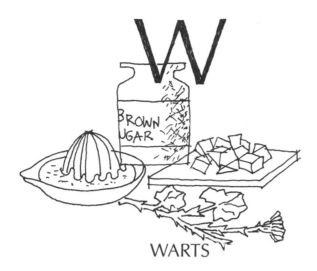

WARTS

These are small benign tumours arising from the outer layers of the skin. They are caused by a contagious virus which causes a wart to form on susceptible people.

Preventative: Thuja 30c taken once a week for a month can remove the personal susceptibility to warts.

LEMON JUICE can help remove hard skin.

CASTOR OIL if applied day and night, should remove the wart slowly.

CELANDINE JUICE, DANDELION SAP, THUJA TINCTURE OR CREAM AND TEA-TREE OIL applied directly to the wart can help remove it.

WATER RETENTION
(see Dropsy)

DANDELION, YARROW OR BEARBERRY TEAS taken in combination or separately, can help remove excess water from the body tissues.

WHIPLASH

This is the injury suffered when a vehicle is hit hard from the rear, forcing the head to jerk violently forward and then backwards, causing injury.

These remedies can be taken once every day for two weeks:

HYPERICUM 30c can be used for nerve pain and damage.

COCCUS CACTI 30c is for a paroxysmal cough with much discharge.

WORMS

There are three common types of worm: threadworms, roundworms and tapeworms.

Threadworms are the most common. They are around twelve mm in length. The eggs are laid around the anus. Symptoms include irritability, itching anus, burning nose, and worms in the stool. Good hygiene, including washing hands, wearing clean underwear and clean bedding, is crucial. Roundworms occur in most parts of the world, though they cause few symptoms except a cough or weight loss.

These remedies can be used for threadworms and roundworms:

OLIVE OIL rubbed around the anus means that the worms find it difficult hold onto the skin.

ONIONS, GARLIC, PICKLES AND SALT all provide an unpleasant internal environment for the worms.

WORMWOOD TEA, TANSY TEA OR QUASSIA TEA canbe taken three times a day for three or four days. Wormwood tea can work exceptionally well though it has a very bitter taste.

NAT-PHOS 6c taken three times daily for two weeks can help to create a hostile environment for worms.

These remedies can be taken three times daily for three days and repeated in three days', time if symptoms still remain:

CHINA 30c can be useful when there is an itching anus, itching and burning nose, grinding teeth, irritability, dark rings under the eyes, and sleep loss.

TEUCRIUM 30c can be useful when there is much rectal itching and sleep loss.

Tapeworms are caused by eating infected pig's meat, however, they are very rare in the West.

PUMPKIN SEEDS made into a paste with honey, and taken for three or four days, can help remove the worm.

CASTOR OIL by the spoonful three times daily should clear the worms.

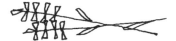